THOUGH THE MOUNTAINS BE SHAKEN

Written by
Ariel Selwyn

ISBN: 978-1-7347115-0-9
Copyright Registration: 1-8585285251

Dedication

"To my four bundles of joy, Tyler, Audrey, Connor, and Karis, and to my supportive husband, Matt."

Contents

Contents

Foreword

Most people speak of war and its ravages on countries and their people in stark terms, understanding what they see and read in the daily broadcasts. Likewise, discussion of diseases and their ravages on the human body are understood, most often with a degree of sympathy with the victim of, say, cancer or HIV/AIDS. However, individuals suffering from tick-borne diseases do not enjoy even a small fraction of the same sympathy or support needed. Often family members dismiss the apparent severity of symptoms and the subsequent degree of disability imposed on those suffering from Lyme alone, and even worse when Lyme is combined with other tick-borne infections like Bartonella, Babesia (a parasite), RMSF, Anaplasma, or Ehrlichia or any combinations of these. Seen from this perspective, the lack of public awareness of the severity of these devastating diseases is almost but not quite understandable.

A corkscrew-shaped bacterial spirochete named *Borrelia burgdorferi* is the cause of Lyme. This spirochete is transferred from an infected tick to the bitten individual without the individual being the wiser. The longer the tick attachment the more likely it will transmit pathogens it carries. Not all ticks harbor infections, of course, but this depends on many factors and geographic amenities. Some ticks harbor and can transmit multiple infections during a single bite.

Lyme disease is a world-wide epidemic, not only a US-based disease. Lyme is the twenty-first century great imitator, mimicking a large variety of illnesses such as Chronic Fatigue Syndrome, Fibromyalgia, migraines, chronic neck pain, palpitations, joint pain and swelling or various psychiatric manifestations. It affects all organs of the body, invading the tissue, causing damage and triggering inflammation. Its favorite destinations are joints, the heart and nervous systems. Delay in

1

diagnosis (usually due to misdiagnosis) and delay in treatment allows the damage to progress unchecked. By invading lymph nodes and lymphatic system, Lyme suppresses the immune system further wreaking havoc, allowing a surge of dormant or previously contained infections to flourish unheeded. Examples of the later include Mycoplasma, Chlamydia, dysentery, Coxsakie virus, Herpes class viruses such as HSV-I, HSV-II, HHV6, CMV, or fungi/mold, or parasites such as protozoa, helminths and filaria. Chemicals add to this toxic mixture as do heavy metals.

Those unfortunate individuals who either had inadequate initial treatment or delay of diagnosis suffer from a very poor health related life quality. It is estimated that this group represent thirty-five to forty-five percent of those diagnosed with Lyme. This group of individuals with chronic Lyme suffer worse fatigue than those with congestive heart failure for instance. Pain and fatigue is disabling and draining. Other manifestation pile on, including exhaustive fatigue, insomnia or excess sleepiness that does not respond to prolonged sleep, whole body pain, joint pain, muscle achiness, cognitive impairment, nerve pain, headaches, palpitations, anxiety, panic and depression. Chronic Lyme signs, symptoms and pathologic findings are exactly the same as late (tertiary) syphilis, another devastating spirochetal bacterium. The mainstream medical community still vehemently argues against the possibility of the B. burgdorferi spirochete persistence causing chronic Lyme but they accept the chronicity of syphilis.

A patient-conceived and powered research project known as MyLymeData allows patients to learn and help each other improve their lives. A MyLymeData survey revealed that sixty-five percent of individuals with chronic Lyme disease cut back or quit work or school and twenty-five percent are disabled. The survey results revealed that about sixty percent reported delay in diagnosis of two or more years, thirty percent were denied insurance coverage of claims and about 60 percent never had a rash or recalled a tick bite. Forty percent saw more than 5 physicians before being diagnosed with Lyme, and thirty percent saw ten or more physicians. Thirty percent have Lyme and Babesia, about thirty percent have Lyme and Bartonella and about 45 percent had Lyme for at least 10 years.

The mainstream medical community – and especially those institutionalized in large hospital, universities and research centers– adds to the suffering by failing to diagnose, properly treat, or even recognize the complexity of the symptoms displayed by Lyme and tick-borne disease patients. It follows that they also fail to recognize the complex therapies needed by such individuals. Indeed, most of these physicians' decree that the patients have an incurable mental illness, or simply prescribe powerful and addicting painkillers. To add to this injustice there is a group of scientist and researchers that sneer and laugh at the suffering of patients with tick-borne disease. This group of supposedly professional resort to name-calling, publishing articles down-playing patients' symptoms, downplaying the research and go out of their way to disprove the persistence and chronicity of Lyme and other tick-borne diseases. They offer their services as expert witnesses, always against patients.

The reality is that all tick-borne illnesses, despite the fact that they come from a tiny tick, afflict people very differently. The ravages on the human body are very personal. Each person experiences a unique set of symptoms pattern based on how their body reacts to the infection, the degree of inflammation induced by the infection(s), the presence of latent previously controlled infections and whether the immune system becomes over-reactive and turns against the body leading to an autoimmune disease. The psychological response by the person is also unique. Any one of tick- borne organisms can be disabling, but they often appear as multiple pathologic organisms, joining forces to affect a lifelong suffering, rapid aging, an almost dehumanizing impact, often sapping the will to live. Tick-borne diseases do not follow the old axiom that one disease state or infection should adequately explain a patient's presentation.

Most evidence shows that these disease agents persist for years, sometimes remaining dormant until activated by stress, major surgery, trauma, steroids or a new infection comes along that suppresses the immune system. All individuals with a history of tick-bites, even those who underwent the mainstream medical community's "adequate treatment" will suffer from symptoms, probably throughout their lives. These viruses, parasites, bacteria can lay dormant for months, years, even decades, and may return to cause more medical problems. Untreated infections are worse, leading to problems such as early onset dementia, Alzheimer's, autoimmune problems, cancer, blood pressure issues, intractable headaches, multi-level spinal stenosis, congestive heart disease, chronic renal failure, gait disturbances, fractures at "decent" bone densities, etc., etc. These "bugs" permeate the body, and their capacity to cause damage is unsurpassed.

All of these "bugs" manifest as inflammation, a fact that the mainstream medicine physicians took too long to understand. Difficult to control or multisystem inflammations generally indicate the presence of an aggressive infection or a combination of infections. Any rheumatologist that understands the problems presented by inflammation should be able to define the root causes of autoimmune diseases. For decades, individuals suffering from tick-borne diseases and related symptoms suffered at the hands of physicians who blamed the symptoms on the process of autoimmune disorder instead of a persistent underlying cause be it infections or increased chemical/heavy metal burden. It took a long time for physicians to understand what was going on; decades of observation by many astute physicians involved in functional medicine unmasked the idea of identifying the infectious root causes of the problem, and therefore also identifying the best means of treating the multiple manifestations inflammation brought on by tick-borne diseases.

Children and teenagers suffer the most at the hands of the mainstream medical community, as their symptoms are mis-identified as psychological issues, or passed off as "normal teenager behavior". There is a grain of truth here, as the diseases lead to many social, psychological, psychiatric and neurocognitive damage. But the root cause is a tick-borne infection, a fact ignored by the mis-diagnosing physician. There are many examples, but one serves to illustrate. I have observed among my younger patients an increase in the practice of "cutting," attributed by other physicians as one or another psychiatric issue like bipolar or obsessive compulsive disorder. When treated for the underlying parasitic infection (such as Babesia, Giardia, Trichinella, or Ascaris roundworm), the tendency and need to cut is completely resolved, and the practice stops.

The mainstream medical community has operated on the idea that 14-28 days of antibiotic therapy is sufficient to cure all tick-borne diseases, despite the preponderance of documentation throughout the world to the contrary. The one-size-fits all approach to medicine is clearly failing in the treatment of all chronic diseases and certainly does not stand up to the complexity of Lyme and a very quickly expanding group of tick transmitted infections. The standard "cookie-cutter" treatments currently recommended does not and will never fix this conundrum. Antibiotics alone are not sufficient in healing those patients with persistent infection. One of the overwhelming issues is the suppression of the immune system by invading pathogens damaging the germinal center of lymph nodes throughout the body. This is the center of the immune system initiation. Clinicians versed in the complexity of the various details of tick-borne infection presentations and tissue damage, and have at their disposal a large armamentarium of conventional and natural therapies are best suited to help patients like Ariel. It takes teamwork and dedication. Physicians specializing in Functional and Integrative Medicine have played a major role in improving the health and wellness of those suffering from persistent Lyme and other tick-borne diseases. These specializations require an exponentially-increasing knowledge and skill, as they seek to optimize all body systems, hormones, glands, mitochondria, immune, intestinal, lymphatic, neurotransmitter, and detoxing systems, seeking to improve the patient's vitality. Often therapies are developed and then abandoned, if the benefits were insufficient to help most patients, while others become cornerstones upon which new therapies can be built. All such therapies must include healthy nutrition, balancing intake of protein and good fats, exercise, lots of water, regular bowel movements, and lots of sunshine. All patients should schedule quiet time and prayer.

Ariel's reflections in this book serve multiple purposes to anyone seeking relief from similar symptoms. The process of recording experiences always helps an individual better understand the disease process, validating those experiences. Further, it allows family and friends to gain a better understanding of the experience and point of view of the patient. A spouse hearing frequently that "I am tired" tends after a while to get used to it, thinking 'so what else is new?' But when a tick-borne disease patient says "I am tired," they frequently mean "my brain is thinking like it's moving through molasses in the cold," or "the pressure in my head feels like its in a vice and may implode any minute," or "I just slept 14 hours straight and feel like sleeping for another 14 hours." A book such as Ariel's may help family or friend to understand this, to get a hint of what the patient is experiencing. Again, teens suffer most from such misunderstanding, as they often seem to be lazy and sullen just because they are teens. If infected, they may in reality be feeling horrible and miserable, and cannot effectively communicate the fact. An understanding parent or friend can be a life-saver. Sadly, and perhaps because of inadequately diagnosed illness, teen cutting is increasing alarmingly, as is also suicide.

Faith, hope, and a good relation with one's Maker are important factors, as seen in Ariel's experience. A crisis of faith is frequently detrimental and difficult to deal with, especially if it combines with low self-esteem or a distorted body image. The loss of all hope is devastating: feeling that God now hates you or is punishing you never leads to a positive outcome, as it causes intense feelings of fear, anxiety, or panic. Judgmental parents, friends, priests or pastors make it hard to adjust one's attitude, and adding to the depth of despair that often accompanies such devastating symptoms. Ariel chose to anchor her faith on John 3:16, the Bible text that points out that God's salvation is not based on one's body of works. It became to her the Rock on which to base her faith, and led eventually to as positive an outcome as is possible.

Perhaps the best contribution of this book is Ariel's journey to health, and her writing of the experience. It demonstrates that life is fragile, a gem in the sun and a light to those around us. I had the privilege of contributing a bit to Ariel's journey; I wish I could have helped more. Life's journey is full of hope and new beginnings. Make every moment count and leave the past in the past. Live each day for its own sake since it is a gift and do not waste the now in living in the past or spending too much time making plans for the future. Most importantly, stay anchored in God's love with his warm comforting arms around you.

L.H. Zackrison, M.D.

Introduction

When the results finally came back, I was at a loss. After spending hours upon hours in the hospital doubled over in excruciating abdominal pain, and undergoing multiple tests, there was no diagnosis for my physical pain. They sent me home with no more answers than I came in with. My experiences were making no sense. Just a short while ago I was a thriving mom, loving the challenge of raising four little ones. I had four healthy pregnancies, lots of energy and was running several miles a day. Then out of nowhere my world started to crumble. My life as I knew it was slipping out of my hands. I had been very good at feeling in control of my life up to this point…or so I thought.

Soon after, in the middle of the night I woke up slammed with a splitting headache. This was nothing new. I had already been dealing with migraines for months. My husband, Matt, was sleeping next to me half awake. I remember thinking, "What if we are in this for the long haul? What would that be like? Could I handle that?" Little did I know it would be a more than 10-year journey of symptom after symptom with no concrete answers. But I was no quitter.

I learned to live with a 24-7 excruciating migraine. I learned to still be a mom with my head feeling like it was going to explode. I had never felt so much pressure in my life. But I refused to let it be my long-term normal. I refused to let it be my forever normal. I learned that I am a lot stronger and more determined than I ever knew. I'm not saying I didn't get discouraged and doubtful many times. But I knew that I would never stop searching for answers, that I would never stop trying.

For 10 years my children watched me struggle to understand the pain, confusion and symptoms that I was experiencing but that no doctor seemed to have a clear answer for. Let me be clear, every specialist thought they had the answer in their area of expertise but what they recommended wasn't taking away the symptoms. Around and around in circles we went. From doctor, back to bed, from invasive test back to the doctor, more medication and back to bed. I kept persevering. Nothing mattered but getting better.

Finally, after being misdiagnosed with things like chronic fatigue syndrome, daily migraines, depression, and IBS, I was diagnosed with chronic Lyme disease and multiple co-infections, as well as an overgrowth of candida, parasites, and more. I was still confused, weary, and wondered if this was really the answer. As Americans we expect quick fixes and when treatment went on for years with no real improvement in symptoms it was difficult and confusing to say the least. My confusion grew stronger and I realized that quick fixes were not the case when it came to late stage chronic Lyme.

The many years that followed were tough. There were endless treatments and tests but I never gave up. I never stopped fighting, and I am thankful for my doctors who never stopped learning and fighting for me. It's a shame that Lyme is so misunderstood and that Lyme specialists are losing their licenses because the VA Board of Physicians only allows Lyme to be treated with three weeks of antibiotics.

During my illness, I felt so guilty and inadequate for not being the wife and mom that I thought I was supposed to be and that I no longer could be. The old me loved to take on more than I could handle and loved the challenge of raising my four little ones, who were 5 and under when it all started. Being a mom was my identity, so losing the ability to enjoy every aspect of being a mom and instead having to grit my teeth through every soccer game and other events and sometimes even miss important milestones was heartbreaking.

Before my symptoms began I felt like I could do anything and I loved life. I felt like it was taken right out from under me in a moment's notice. I was adamant that I would never surrender to this illness, that I would never give up. I always had hope that I would get my life back.

I don't pretend to have all the answers, or any answers for that matter. I am just a mom who has gone through challenges in life, like everyone else, and who has been trying to find my way. I will always be trying to find my way to the best of my abilities. If what I have been through, or what I share, can help someone else, that will make me happy and it will all be worth it.

I am not a doctor and I don't prescribe, diagnose, or treat any illness or disease. Please work with your doctor to find the best treatment options for you.

Prologue

I was dozing off in my room in my hot-pink bean-bag chair and heard a loud knock at the door. I thought it was the kids next door calling for my younger siblings as they often did. I was engaged at the time, still living at home, and had just graduated from the University of Mary Washington in Fredericksburg, Va. I ignored the knocking. It didn't stop and I kept ignoring it thinking it would stop once they realized my siblings weren't home. Over and over again the repeated loud knocking and I was getting annoyed, as I was trying to take a quick power nap. Eventually, it subsided. I ultimately dozed off thinking nothing more of it. A while later I got dressed, packed up my bag, and headed out. I don't remember where I was going but that isn't important. When I opened the door there was a note in familiar handwriting. "I heard you were engaged. Tell him he's a lucky guy." Omigod. Was it him? I got a pit in my stomach, a heaviness in my chest and stopped dead in my tracks. There was no way I was going anywhere. I had dated someone really special for about a year and a half in high school and early college. I hadn't wanted to break up with him. I showed it to my stepdad, Dan. Instead of talking it through with me he grabbed it harshly out of my hand, crumpled it up, and said, "Don't ever think of that again." The sad thing is I didn't think this was abnormal until later in life. The next day or so when I picked up the phone and my neighbor was on the phone with my mom (yes, corded phones) I quickly asked, "Did you see a car in the driveway!?" I was still wondering if there had been any sign of him.

My mom quickly reminded me: "Dan said never to think of it again!" in a firm tone. I slinked back and pushed it out of my mind.

This would come back to haunt me for years to come. Why *hadn't* I stood up for myself? Why HADN'T I thought about it again? Why *didn't* I take the time to decide what I wanted to do with that note or how I wanted to respond to it? Why? Because I didn't know how to think for myself. I hadn't been taught to think for myself. And I regret it. I regret all those years of not thinking for myself. It's hard not to blame myself. But it's all I knew. Even to this day as a 40-year-old woman, thinking back to that incident is like a punch in the stomach because it reminds me of how over-protective, though probably well-meaning, my mother and stepdad were and makes me question, Did I even choose my life? Not only in that instance but altogether. And it makes me sad. I fault myself often for not standing up for myself. For not knowing how, for not listening to my dad when he said they were "brainwashing" me. They were so good at it, so good at making me believe they were right.

It wasn't until I was an adult, after a long run, standing in the driveway of our King George house, that I had a meltdown realizing my life had not been my own. I thought back to the note and I wished I had had the confidence to tell my stepdad that it was mine, and taken a moment to think about it and consider what I wanted to do with it. Actually, I wish I had had parents who would have encouraged me more to think for myself and asked me, "What do YOU think? What do YOU want to do?"

I thought back to when my parents left the church that I had grown up in. That church was my home. It was my life. I was living at home at the time but attending UMW, where I studied and ultimately graduated with a B.S. in mathematics. I wish I had had the notion to say that I'm old enough to make my own decisions and I want to stay in this church that is my home instead of following them without question because I was "under their authority" as they had taught us. But that is what I was taught, to follow them. No questions asked. Or I was "opening myself to the Devil" if I disobeyed. My mom and stepdad did what they thought was best as parents, but they came from a different world and mind set, and could not fully understand my emotional needs.

This wondering what my life would have been if I had only stood up more for myself would go on to haunt me even through my adult years. This would drive me back to therapy.

My mother and stepdad were a part of a group called ATI, Advanced Training Institute. Looking back, it held for me a very restrictive view of life. ATI put the Bible into a lot of steps. For example, if you want forgiveness, follow these five steps. The most significant piece of training that affected our family was their teaching that the children were under an umbrella of authority (the father) and if you didn't obey what the father said, you were giving ground to the enemy, who was Satan. You can imagine the fear that instilled in me. As a result I believed in only obeying and doing what my stepdad decided as opposed to thinking for myself. This gave no room for my own decisions or choices. I remember my birth father saying that they were overly controlling me, but again I didn't realize it because it was just the way that I grew up. Looking back, I was mad at myself for not being able to be my own person and stand up for myself, but as my best friend, Stephanie, told me when we were growing up, we instinctively trust our parents and learn from them, so she encouraged me not blame myself.

When it came to college, thankfully I had the grades to get into Mary Washington at the time. Looking back, I wish I had had the confidence to take out loans and go away to college to get out from under my family's influence but I didn't know any better at the time. I had lived in their strict world for too long. I didn't know how to think for myself or that I even could do such a thing. Actually, they probably wouldn't have let me since they were the parents and I was the child.

It would take years of being married and thus out from under their influence to realize how restrictive was my upbringing. It would take most of my adult life to learn who Ariel was, to learn how to be my own person. I didn't morph into the true Ariel overnight. It is still taking time. I still see remnants of my parents in me and have to change my way of thinking and ask myself what do I think. Because of that, I believe one of the biggest gifts I can give my children is to believe in who they are as an individual, to tell them I not only love them but that I am proud of them just the way they are.

Maybe we all have regrets, but I wish I would've been able to see back then what I can see now.

****

You can imagine that I grew up in a very strict but what my family thought was a well-meaning household. I lived with my mother, stepdad, two half-sisters and a half-brother. I visited my dad and stepmom, Debbie, and other brother and sister several times a week, and for that occasional change I am very grateful for the breathing space.

Although I believe they were trying to do their best, growing up with my mom and stepdad left no room for Grace. This is where my deep-rooted belief of never being good enough originated. I couldn't even shake in it adulthood. My mother was and is not very open-minded because of her upbringing and station in life, and my stepdad was a very serious man much of my younger years. My birth father has a way of sarcastically joking with a little truth behind it. Although I always tried to let it roll off my shoulders, the little bit of always poking fun and the sometimes tone of disapproval affected me. However, it was my mom and stepdad's too high standards, frequent judgment, and over-protection that really influenced my poor frame of mind. Because of that, to this day, I still struggle with feelings of not feeling good enough.

16

I remember my mom and stepdad joking that we deserved death. What they meant was that because of mankind's sin we deserved death. Which was true...our sin separated us from God and we no longer had eternal life (without Jesus). But really, that described their root beliefs — more focus on death instead of life. More focus on sin instead of God's Grace and Mercy. More focus on rules and rigidity and what we were doing wrong than what God did for us when He sent His son, Jesus. This was their heart-felt religious view of life, what they believed in, and the only way they know how to live their lives.

It wasn't until I was an adult and away from that home life long enough that I could see the difference. I remember one day when my mom in her life-long religious mind set said to my youngest, "You know, we deserve death," that I softened that comment with, "NO! No, we don't. We deserve everything that Jesus does." We deserve life. Why? Because we are covered in the blood of Jesus. We look like Jesus to God, holy, blameless, righteous, and perfect NOW. All because of what Jesus did on the cross. And because of that, when we mess up, we can up and try again. We don't have to wallow in guilt and shame. That was what the missing part of the religious message when I grew up. I wallowed in guilt and shame. I needed the life part, the Grace part, the Mercy part.

It wasn't until I was an adult that I knew that God rejoices over us with singing. (Zephania 3:17)

That means that now I can pull off and let go of what I felt were all the chains and burdens of being crushed by beliefs of not being good enough and feeling like a failure because I am perfect and holy and righteous in Christ now already, even while He is still making me more like Jesus.

I didn't grow up in a home that always portrayed this Grace. This Grace side of God was often missing. I grew up with the obedience side of God. The rules side of God. But I also needed the Grace and love side.

Their way of thinking was ingrained in me into adulthood. I didn't know how to be myself, without the burdens and chains. I didn't know how to be Ariel with God's love and grace. I didn't know how to be Ariel with an open mind until years and years of living on my own. It was what they thought was best in molding me. I found it easier to comply than to risk getting into trouble. After years and years of being away from their home I would finally learn who the real Ariel was and learn that Ariel was good enough.

****

One of the most painful things in my life was not always feeling I had my own mother's full support. But then what child doesn't always feel that way? When I suffered through an eating disorder and a chronic illness my mother believed in her faith that it was from sin in my life. This affected me with guilt and shame. It seemed to be part of my mother and stepdad's personality and nature because of their beliefs that criticism and judgment were productive. There is already a lot of guilt and shame that comes with an eating disorder, thus I felt like more of a failure. My mom and stepdad were the parents who rarely said, "I'm proud of you." They were the kind who corrected you and told you where you could improve so that you could be a better person. They truly believed that. But I guess many a child would also see their parents as being that way. This way of parenting unfortunately did not mesh well with my personality. I needed encouragement. Instead of becoming strong under their criticism, a solid, deep-rooted belief of not being good enough in any area of my life took root.

During my college years and beyond, not only did my mother tell me my eating disorder was a sin, but she was not as supportive as I would want her to be when my health spiraled downward. She lived in my neighborhood right down the street and around the corner but was unable in her mind set to always feel my need. Faced with the same situation, I would like to think that if any of my kids went through what I went through I would be over at their house doing their laundry, cleaning their house, taking care of their kids, running their errands, doing whatever they needed. Did I expect that of her? No, not at all. I'm a very self-sufficient independent person. But because of her ways, she didn't do any of that. But I DID think she could have, should have been able to support me emotionally. But she didn't or just wasn't able to. She was judging me for the doctors I was seeing, she was telling me that my health struggles were from sin in my life. Of course, that's what she was taught to believe. At one point through my health journey there was a man in our church going through cancer treatment. Would she tell him his cancer was from sin? I don't think so, but the difference, of course I had to realize, was because he was not her child. But my health struggles were from sin. Go figure. She was helping another elderly lady in the area, but she wasn't helping me as much as I wanted her to, in the ways that I needed her. I remember finding out that she was helping the lady and crying, wondering why she wasn't there for me, when I was floundering. I wasn't asking for the world. I just wanted positive emotional support, if that makes sense. Perhaps I should have reached out more and told her how much more, or the kind of support I needed.

My mother is all about conventional doctors, so I stopped telling her about any alternative practitioners whom I was seeing. Everyone is entitled to their own opinion, but I needed my mom to care more about what I felt I needed medically. I needed her to care about me. I needed her support. I was already floundering and struggling both physically and emotionally. I didn't need her judgment; I just needed a mom. I was just doing the best I could to take care of my kids and try to get better. My stepmom would always keep my doctor's appointments straight and ask me the latest update, but my mom? She did not always think to ask. It was her way, but it hurt.

I remember at Matt's and my wedding my dad gave a very touching and loving speech that meant so much to me. My mom said, "Oh, I knew Dad would take the opportunity to look good in front of all those people from our past." She meant that in her mind he'd put the time and effort into the speech to redeem himself in front of them, and not to honor me. It hurt that she would take that from me when she knew that I'd had so many insecurities from my parents' divorce. At least, that's the way it seemed to me now and at the time. Again, it's just her way.

One bright sunny day I was sitting in the parking lot of my Ear Nose and Throat Doctor. I was on the phone with my mother catching up on life. I mentioned to her that my sister (on my Dad's side) got a new roommate. He happened to be gay. Let me just say here that this was my sister's best friend and I absolutely love this friend of hers and he has been an amazing friend to her. My mom gasped and said, "What is she going to do if he brings someone home!!??" I was shocked and dumbfounded. I didn't respond at all. But I was thinking, "Nothing. Nothing mom, because no one cares about that but you." This was an example of the ways of thinking that I had to peel off. This was the kind of judgment that I grew up with.

When my sister and step mother went over to my mother's house to help with wedding decorations for mine and Matt's wedding, my mother hurt my sister to her very core. They were in the kitchen alone and my mother mentioned that it was going to be harder for my sister to find someone to get her dress made because of her weight. She went on to say that it didn't have to be that way because healthy food tastes good too. She asked my sister if she was going to go on a diet for the wedding. This was the first time that my sister realized she was overweight and it still brings her to tears to this day even in her thirties. She was twelve at the time

It took years of being away from them for my eyes to be opened and to, one step at a time, start shedding their way of thinking and start figuring out who I was, who Ariel was. I was angry at first but I have become more accepting of it now. I just want to be open minded and figure out who I am and how I think.

I know that relationships aren't perfect. We can't expect them to be and we can't expect to get all we need emotionally from everyone. However, it's important that we learn to be at peace with what happened and realize we can't change it. I think my mother was the best mom she knew how to be. She has her own pain and scars. She may not have had the emotional ability to give much. I don't really know. She may have had her own insecurities. I know my dad had an unusual and rough past, and he was the best dad that he knew how to be, and I can give him Grace and I need to extend that same Grace toward my mother. However, that doesn't mean I don't also wish I had more of the support that I feel I need from her. I know that because who she is, she can't help herself from being critical. Thus, I have to learn to have a relationship with her that I feel comfortable with because I need and want her in my life and in my children's lives. I'm not sure what that full relationship is yet, and it may change and evolve to look different at different times in my life. Right now I need space in order to protect myself.

I see other mom-and-daughter relationships and how giving those moms are and I will be honest, I am jealous because I would like the same. I wonder why my mother isn't what I feel should be more giving like that. Maybe she doesn't have the emotional ability to give of herself. And that's OK. Everyone is different and everyone has to care for themselves. I honestly don't think she realized when she was being too critical of me. I think it was part of her nature. She loves me the best way she can but I feel she doesn't know how to be proud of me. Maybe she just wasn't able to give me the emotional support that I needed, and I have to accept the kind of mom that I have and not long for something different.

Maybe I have to learn to be able to do that with all of my past. To be at peace with what happened, to accept it and not long for something else, because I don't think I'm there yet with parts of my past. I'm not pretending to give advice here. I'm not pretending to have answers. I'm a huge work in progress. I just want others to know that they aren't alone. That I'm wondering, processing, living, and growing with you.

It's not a secret that my current relationship with my mother at the time of this writing is strained. I found that every time we talked she said something that I interpreted as hurtful and critical. Perhaps she didn't really mean it that way. Matt would tell me to brush it off, that she's never going to change, so just accept it. I tried but it would eat away at me, even when I went back to work full time and it was a HUGE transition in my life physically, emotionally, and mentally. As I left the kids after 15 years of being home, she didn't think to ask me how it was going and it's been a full year now as I'm writing this book. A full year that she's had a chance to ask me how it's going. Wouldn't you also think that a normal question for a mom to ask? Eventually, around 38/39 years old I decided I didn't need judgy, critical people in my life anymore. I wanted to surround myself with my friends who were supportive and encouraging and who were my true friends. So, I've resorted to only texting my mother when I had to. Maybe I will regret it one day because in the long run everyone needs their mom. I just don't need that negativity in my life anymore. The kids even picked up on it and asked at times, "Mom, why isn't Adee always nice to you?" They call her Adee.

Recently, though, my mother has started to try but it's hard to believe she will change the only way she knows how to be. She tries to be encouraging in a birthday card or a Mother's Day card, for example, but I find it hard to accept that. After years and years of being judged and criticized I can't take encouraging words from her without some doubt whether she can be the mom I would like her and need for her to be. Maybe one day but not now.

In raising my kids, I wanted to break the cycle of my former home life and have a more open mind with my kids. I love to show excitement to see my kids and tell them that I love to spend time with them, tell them I am proud of them and that they can do anything they want. I let my kids have a lot of freedom and that allows me to have a relationship with them. You can't have a relationship with your kids if you control them. You can't have a relationship with your kids if you are hovering over them and smothering them.

I remember getting to know my Uncle Tommy and Aunt Cathy better as I got older and thinking these are my favorite people in the whole world because they are so open minded and so NON-judgmental.

My mom and stepdad used to be wary of them because they felt they were not disciplining their kids the same way that they did. However, I was able to see the good relationship that they were able to have with their kids. And to me that is very important.

When we were growing up I had to listen to my mother and step father criticize our extended family, families in our church and even the elders of our church. When you are little, you think your parents must be right. I had to become an adult and get to know my family and church family for myself and realize they are truly wise and amazing people. I was angry at first. I was angry that they led us to believe false views of others. But I had to accept that they must have been dealing with their own insecurities

I know I have shared some harsh words. All in all, I do believe my parents were trying their best like most parents do. I believe they thought they were doing the right thing. It's just unfortunate that I felt it was hurtful in the long run.

I'm sure my kids will grow up and say I did this or that wrong and I will have to apologize. I am far from being perfect. I worry about not spending enough time with my kids. I worry about if I am doing something to mess them up. I worry about what they will blame me for. I worry. Worry. worry...but I do want to learn from the mistakes of my mother and stepdad and leave what I saw were the critical and restrictive ways far behind.

Last night as I was getting ready for bed, as I was lying down I felt a healing toward my mother. I thought for a split second maybe I should let her back in. Honestly I don't feel any bitterness towards my mother or stepfather. I certainly don't want the bitterness in my heart. It's no good for me. And I know that forgiveness doesn't mean we forget. I want to be kind but I have been in this place before where I am afraid to let her too close because every time I fear she will continue to be hurtful again. I mean she was just critical this last spring when I had to be around her for the kids' soccer game. I brought up that I might have to travel for work and she said without thinking, "Well if it were me I would do the least travel as possible." And I just know behind that she's thinking that because I'm a mom I should be home as much as possible. It's a little dig in my mind. Whenever she takes digs at me I can't ever think in the moment. And I wish I would have stood up for myself and said, "Well then I wouldn't be the best. And I want to be the best." I always want to be the best at whatever I do and work is no different. I know that when we were younger, my stepdad gave up opportunities at work because he didn't want to travel. But overall, I think that they could have taught us to think big and learn how to live outside their bubble. They didn't teach us to go after our dreams. Now, I'm not saying that my job is my dream. But what I AM saying is that I have had to learn to think big and to go after my dreams and to teach my kids to go after their dreams. And I can work and travel with work AND be a good mom. I have had to figure it out and still am trying to figure it out, but there is no need to take a dig at me. That is just her way, I know, and my husband, Matt, is right--she will never change. I believe I wouldn't ever take digs at my kids.

So, after all that, I may have felt my heart changing a bit to my mother but I am always apprehensive of what I see as more criticism and that is the reason I distanced myself from her. But I am thankful that God has taken away the bitterness. As I was driving in the car the other day, some questions came to mind. Do I need to repair the relationship with my mom? I don't always want to because I am afraid she will hurt me over again like in the past. But maybe I am supposed to repair the relationship, expecting her to hurt me and just forgive her over and over and over just like Jesus forgives me over and over and over. It's confusing. I mean, I know I have to forgive her time and time again. But do I have to put myself in the position to be hurt?

Why can I forgive my mother? Because her hurt/sin against me is not between her and me. It's between her and God. Who am I to judge? God is the only judge. If I don't/can't forgive her I am saying Jesus is not enough for her sins. God poured out His wrath upon Jesus for her sins just as he poured out His wrath upon Jesus for my sins and Jesus absorbed them all. Therefore, they are over and done with. And I can move on. It's between her and God.

25

Like I said, I believe my mother is trying to change in some areas. Now that I have gone back to work she is being supportive in her way by picking the kids up two days a week to take them to the pool or bowling. But the thing is, I don't need her that much now. The kids are older. That's fine if she wants to pick them up, but they would also be fine if she didn't. I needed her more back then. I needed her more when the kids were little and I was ill. I needed her to support me more and not judge me and not make me feel like I owed her when she watched my kids. That's why I started taking them to all the doctor's appointments with me. I needed her support more when I was in college and was struggling with an eating disorder. But I can't blame her for who she was/is. I don't want to judge her because that's not whom I want her to be. She was/is who she is and good for her for trying to change. It's a shame it all comes back to that I just don't trust her to not hurt me again. I can forgive her over and over, but I have to use common sense. And I don't want to put myself in a place where I have to be criticized over and over. It just doesn't make sense.

Over the years I thought that I had seen some glimpses of change in them. I hoped I was right. However, when I was blessed with a. modeling opportunity they were unable to be happy for me. They immediately said it was a scam and not legitimate. It unfortunately reminded me that they had the same critical spirit towards me.

Again, I don't share any of this to bash my mother and step father. In fact, when I have brought up any of this to them, 95% of it they deny and say that I am distorted in my thinking. It's really sad. My step father has implied that I am a liar and refused to apologize when my supportive husband has asked him to. I don't think they are harming the relationship maliciously. I think it's just who they are. It's sad because over the years I have thought that I have seen glimpses of them changing. However, things like these are big red flags that they are still the same people that are refusing to grow.

I wanted to mention here that I know a lot of people struggle with way worse family relationships than I have. So many people have had WAY worse childhoods than I had. I am so grateful that I had parents and stepparents who really did love me and I believe tried to do their best. I wasn't physically or sexually abused or anything else horrible that so many others experience, and I have two friends whose mothers were maliciously mean to them. What I want to say to those of you who have gone through any kind of pain whether big or small is that God is ALWAYS protecting us. I know it is hard to see sometimes and it is so often hard to understand, but one thing that has helped me in healing is to pray specifically asking God to give me a visual of where He was during a specific painful moment. Where was He when such and such was happening, and He always shows me. He always answers me. He is always there protecting me. We may not fully understand the entire big picture but He promises never to leave us or forsake us and He is true to His promises.

I also don't want to judge my mother and stepdad and I don't want to be critical. I sat down and asked God to give me a heart of gratitude and to show me the positive things in my childhood. I believe my mother loved me as a little girl. They love my kids. They let my oldest, Tyler, buy one of their cars for a really good deal. I know they love spending time with their grandkids. We always had family dinners together. That is an area I lack in as a parent. My mother has said she is sorry for saying the eating disorder was sin in my life. They have said they are sorry for the way ATI hurt me and my siblings. I am not saying they are horrible people. No parents are perfect. I remember them making time for me to stay up late and talk in college. I just think they didn't know any better. Nevertheless, it left pain that I had to deal with. I know God is in control and He's not throwing His hands in the air saying, "Oh, no, how did Ariel end up with these parents?" Nope. He is using it to make me more like Christ. So, it is good.

****

My parents divorced just before I turned 4 and both parents remarried by the time I was 5 and 6. Although I lived with my mom and stepdad, my dad, lived nearby and was always a part of my life. I was always so grateful that he didn't just up and leave never to be seen again. He was always the best dad he knew how to be under the circumstances.

I don't remember the divorce but my mom says I was playing outside and my dad told me. She says that I came in to her and was upset. She could tell that my dad had said something to me and I said something like, "I don't want Dad to move away."

My dad lived nearby after the divorce and always picked me up one weekday a week and every other weekend. I thought it was normal. I mean, other kids' parents got divorced. I really didn't think it affected me. I was thankful that my dad was in my life and he always told me that he left my mom, not me.

I didn't realize until college that the divorce had indeed affected me. I was sitting in a study room at UMW and I just started welling up inside. I knew tears were coming and I had no idea why. I rushed out of the building and ran to my car as fast as I could. I balled all the way home and I still had no idea why I was crying. My mom asked me what was wrong as I burst through the door. Then it came out of nowhere: "I HATE that you and Dad are divorced." There is was.

That opened up a floodgate of emotions, thoughts, and feelings that I never knew were there. I had a long talk with my dad about feeling like I had missed out on growing up with him and that he had a different relationship with my sister and brother from him and my stepmom and a stronger bond with them. He listened and understood but there was nothing he could do about it. Nevertheless, it was a good conversation and I felt better.

That didn't take away all the other realizations swirling around in my head. I always felt stuck in the middle. I never felt fully part of either family. I wasn't a full part of my mom and stepdad's family. My mom remarried when I was 6 and started having baby after baby after baby in her new life. I didn't even have the same last name. I know she loved me but my stepdad wasn't my dad, and I always resented him for trying to take on that authoritative place in my life when my dad was still in the picture.

I wasn't a full part of my dad and stepmom's family because, for one, I didn't live with them. I was only there a few days a week. That wasn't my home. Where was my home? I knew everyone loved me but where did I really fit in? Plus, it was like two different worlds. I had my legalistic mom and stepdad on one side and my open-minded and worldly dad and stepmom on the other. I'd have to re-adjust my brain going from one house to the other. Not to mention I was a people pleaser. Let's face it. Yes, lots of people get divorced, so it seems like a normal thing these days. But it's not. Divorce is not natural. And it's the kids who suffer the most. My heart always aches for the kids.

I struggled through feelings over the divorce into adulthood. It was weird. Even though I loved all my siblings SO much and I loved my stepmom and stepdad and was thankful for them, there was this little tiny piece deep down that wished my mom and dad had stayed together. It was like that was how it was supposed to be. There was pain there even though I had never known them to be together. My mom had mentioned something about the ring that my dad had given her, and I asked if she still had it and she snapped, "Why would you want

THAT!?" Because that would have been really special to me to have the ring that MY dad gave to MY mom. She couldn't understand it. When my sister eventually got married, her husband's parents were divorced, and he didn't seem to have a problem with it. My mother said to me, "Yeah, you know, he just lets it roll off of him, unlike people like you." I wasn't trying to make it hard. I didn't know I was going to have all these pushed-down emotions well up to the surface in college and early adulthood. I'm sorry Mom, I was trying to cope with them.

As an adult with kids I decided it wasn't my job to make everyone comfortable. It wasn't my problem anymore that I was in the middle between two families. It wasn't my problem to please everyone. I wasn't going to have separate birthday parties for my kids. They would have to get over it and be around each other. For the most part, they do a good job. Everyone is cordial. My stepmom is the sweetest and makes everyone feel welcome and comfortable.

As I got older my relationship with my dad got better. My stepmom has always been a friend and I appreciate that she never tried to take the place of my mom. She was just there for me.

I don't remember much of my early years. I never remember my mom and dad together other than a fight they had. All I remember about that fight is my mom in the bathroom doing her hair and my dad yelling.

I don't have many memories of being young when my mom and stepdad first got married other than playing football in the back yard with my stepdad and reading *Little House on the Prairie* with my mom. I do remember accepting Jesus into my heart with my mom when I was 6. I was in the kitchen with her making something to eat and I remember at that time being more worried about not going to hell than anything else!

30

* *

I went to Battlefield Middle School for third and fourth grade. Battlefield didn't have walls, so the classrooms were very open. My third-grade teacher was Mrs. Carey. She was known to be tough but I made it through. I specifically remember her asking us what our weights were and when me this other little girl and I told her ours she didn't believe us. I had always been very skinny, so my weight was low. I don't know why I remember that.

My fourth-grade teacher was Mr. Sipple. I got in trouble over and over for talking in his class. I had a good friend in his class, Christine. I am friends with her on Facebook today. I had transferred to Battlefield from Lee Hill Elementary, where I attended first through second grade because my mom taught there. When she quit to stay home with my little sister after my second-grade year, I had to start going to the school in the district we were in.

We lived in a green rambler on Green Arbor Drive and I had a dog named Doggy Bear. We didn't have a fence, so he was chained up in the back yard and I would go out and play with him. We moved when I went into fifth grade, into the house I grew up in, and I transferred to Salem Elementary fifth grade. That house was in Fredericksburg, Va., with a split foyer and where I have all my teen and young adult memories. That house is where I first learned to drive, where I snuck out and where I rushed home to try to meet curfew, where I fought with my parents, and where I grew up with my siblings. I had one good friend in that neighborhood, Dusty. When we were in middle school we would play outside together and ride bikes together. We went on a few trips to the mountains together with her family. She was a good friend.

I went to Chancellor Middle School. My best friend, Robyn, and I were inseparable in middle school. We had a blast and I don't know how I'd have gotten through middle school without her. We went to the beach together every summer and were boy crazy, typical middle school girls. I also met my current best friend, Stephanie, in middle school, although we weren't as close then. We grew closer in high school. Unfortunately, Robyn went to Courtland High School and I went to Chancellor High School. I remember my ninth-grade year being very lonely. I had a few friends but wasn't really close with anyone. Robyn and I still got together but I missed her.

In 10th grade, I found a group of friends and in 11th, Stephanie and I bonded for life. By 11th grade I had a good number of friends, all from different groups/clicks. When I look back at high school, I look back with fondness. I enjoyed my high school years. I was on the tennis team, number one seed for my junior and senior years, as well as in the National Honor Society and in multiple clubs.

I went to The University of Mary Washington...mostly because that was my only choice. My parents didn't have money to send me away to school, so my options were to go to the community college nearby or live at home as a commuter at UMW. I was taught to think small. I never would have imagined going out on my own at that point in life. Thinking back, I probably wouldn't have been allowed to. But all in all, it is a very good school and I'm glad I got in.

My college years are some of the loneliest ever but that is not only because I was a commuter. It is because of a hard breakup and mostly because of an eating disorder.

During my college and young adult days I acquired a lot of friends from church and many of them were older adults who served as mentors. I am so thankful for their wisdom in my life. I think of Mrs. Dowell and Mrs. Garbee, Mrs. Bell and Mrs. Hogan. They spoke truth into my life. I still walk regularly with Mrs. Dowell and am so grateful for her friendship. I dove into God's word on my own and through church and Bible studies in college mostly because I was hurting and didn't know where else to turn. I attended several young adult Bible Studies classes.

Chapter 1: Courtship

I remember the day like it was yesterday. When I think about it now, I get this hollow feeling in the pit of my stomach. I never wanted to break up with him. When he left for college he said he loved me to infinity through tears. If I thought him leaving for college was hard, breaking up with him was 1,000 times harder. He made me feel like I was the most special girl in the whole world. I didn't know that when I broke up with him I would not only lose him, but I would lose my whole self I didn't know that when I lost him I would also fall into an eating disorder that would go on for 20 plus years and I would never be the same again.

Leading up to the breakup I kept getting these little hints, I'll call them, from the Lord. At every sermon, every time I would read God's Word, like God was telling me to break up with him, until I couldn't ignore it anymore. I felt 100% sure at the time that God was telling me to break up with him and I was obeying Him. Looking back, I question whether it was my parent's strong influence teaching me that I had to have the certain kind of boyfriend, the certain kind of husband, so I was "hearing" what I thought I was supposed to. Now, being out from under them and thankfully being more open minded I can see that we could have grown together over time, and I regret it. Not just the act itself, but I regret it because of how much control and influence my parents had over me. Nevertheless, I carried out what I thought God was telling me to do at the time. As soon as I broke up with my long-term high school/college boyfriend not only was I a disaster but my parents came across courtship material. I think they read a book or something. I know it was popular in the ATI group they were in. There were families in ATI writing books/testimonies about it. They asked me to commit to it. This meant never dating again, but instead if a guy asked me out, I would have to tell them to go talk to my stepdad. When they went to my stepdad he would then explain to them this courtship idea and that there was no reason to date unless we were of marriageable age and he would offer to disciple them. This took me out of the picture. I think they thought they were doing what was best for me at the time. I think their intention was to protect me from more hurt but really looking back it ended up feeling more controlling and making me feel like it was another thing that wasn't my own, that I didn't make my own decisions.

Remember the whole umbrella of authority and if I went against my God- given authority I was giving ground to the Devil. So, what could I do? I had to say OK. I think at the time I truly didn't want to be hurt so badly again but looking back, I was not sure this was the way to do it. I don't think you can really ever protect your kids from being hurt. You have to do your best and let them live their lives.

There were a handful of guys that came along...these were my college years. I sent them to my stepdad. Some were gone right away (probably scared silly) and some stuck around for a while. I didn't ever get the whole story. When I say stuck around I mean they kept meeting with my stepdad and they were allowed to email me and talk to me in group settings as friends. I never knew what they spoke to my stepdad about and I was to print out any emails between us and put them on my stepdad's dresser so that he could read them. Yes, at the time I thought this was normal and "protection". Looking back, I think it's overly protective to say the least.

It didn't protect me from hurt. Of course, I wondered what was going on between them and when they stopped meeting with my stepdad and stopped talking to me I wondered what had happened. Would it have worked out if my stepdad wasn't involved? Was I not good enough? There were still emotions involved. There always are with girls. You can't completely take that away.

The one that stuck around the longest is obviously Matt, who would be my future husband. We had a calculus class together first semester of freshman year but we never spoke. I remember him riding his bike by me every day freshman year with his blue hat and smiling at me. Although we were both math majors we actually spoke to each other the first t me in Spanish class second semester of freshman year. He approached me freshman year, pretty soon after the breakup actually. I think I actually told him about the breakup if I remembe˙ correctly and told him I wasn't ready for anything for a long time. However, by the end of freshman year he asked if I would want to meet up for lunch over the summer. Ugh, dread. I had to tell him about my stepdad. Matt was a new Christian, so he was a little intrigued by the idea. He was intrigued by my faith as well. He ended up hearing the spiel from my stepdad and realized nothing was going to happen between us for a while. However, the two of them ended up meeting together weekly for years, stucying the Bible. Matt and I stayed friends and he said he stayed interested and "stalked" me, finding out my schedule every semester so that he could "bump" into me. Because we were both math majors we ended up having a lot of classes together.

Once junior year rolled around, he asked my stepdad if we could begin courting. After a week, my stepdad told me he asked. I was surprised and unsure. I was in the worst of my eating disorder and was numb to the idea. I didn't have any feelings at all. My stepdad told Matt it wasn't good timing. I think Matt felt kind of awkward because the next time he saw me he rushed toward me and wanted to talk right away. I didn't feel awkward at all. We took a walk on campus and talked through some things. The summer went by and I started having some feelings toward Matt. The eating disorder was getting a little better as far as my weight coming back up and being stable and I had some time to think things through. I was ready to start "courting" that fall.

Matt came back for school and I expected him to meet with my stepdad, my stepdad tell him I was ready, and we'd start courting. Well, my stepdad told him that I was ready and Matt wasn't expecting it and said he had to think about it. What? I was a basket case at a wedding I was in that weekend and thought he was a huge jerk. Thankfully, he came to his senses over the weekend and was ready. He said he was just caught off guard. So, we started "courting." None of us really knew what that meant.

All we knew was that we were supposed to get to know each other in group settings and/or within the context of each other's families and at the same time be praying about whether we were meant to be together for marriage. We moved forward for months and as Matt got surer, I became unsure. I just wasn't into it. He wanted to spend time together and I didn't. I just didn't have the romantic feelings that I should have had. You can see why, though. This whole process takes a bit of the romance out of it, as I look back. Thankfully, I took a walk with a good friend and as I shared my concerns, she told me, "Matt's not the problem, it's YOU!"

Eventually, I told Matt we needed to talk. We sat downstairs in my parents' basement and I told him I just wasn't sure and I didn't have the feelings and maybe we needed to take a break. I 100% thought that would be it and it would be over. But instead he said OK but he was sure I was the one and he was going to wait for me. Umm, what? OK. Whatever you say, buddy.

Lucky for him, a few days later all the feelings came rushing forward and I was head over heels for Matthew Selwyn. I don't know what did it...maybe what he said...but I just wanted to see him and be with him. I told my mother and step father but they wanted to wait awhile since it was such a big change so fast, but they soon learned that the feelings were here to stay. We actually had a lot of fun once we were both sure. It put some of the butterflies and giddiness back into it.

We still never went out alone until we were engaged and that was less than a handful of times, but we did take walks together and sat outside together and sat on campus together, so it's not like we never had alone time. It just wasn't like we were going out on dates all the time together. He used to bring me hot chocolate and brownies on campus. Very sweet, but yeah he didn't really get the eating disorder yet.

We courted through senior year, nine months to be exact, got engaged right after graduation that spring (May) and got married that coming January. When we look back on our courtship we have a lot of mixed emotions. Matt was a new Christian and was just trying to do things "right," so he went along with it thinking this seemed like a good way to avoid some pitfalls of dating. You already know that I felt like I had to. Was it a bit too much? Yes. Were there some good things about it? Sure. Do I wonder what would have happened if I wasn't doing the courting thing? Of course. Do I wish I'd had more freedom looking back? Yes...in all areas of my life. But it is what it is and I have Matt and I love him and am thankful for him. Will we do this with our kids? Ummm, no.

Do I think there are other ways for people to find their spouse in a godly way? Yes!

Matt and I didn't meet, fall in love, and marry the conventional way, but we made it. We won't put courtship upon our children because that's not who we are. But we also don't think they need to be dating at a super-early age. I think as parents we want what is best for our kids and we want to protect them, and what is most important is seeking the Lord in every step.

Chapter 2: My World Fell Apart

I was a 28-year-old mom loving life. It was 2009. My husband, Matt, and I had four kids in five years. I loved the challenge of it. I loved having them close together and I thought we would have another. I always pictured five. Tyler was 5, Audrey 3, Connor 1 1/2 and Karis 8 months.

I loved being a mom more than anything in the world. Before having kids I taught math at Brooke Point High School in Stafford, Va., for a short period of time. But being a mom was my calling. I loved the midnight feedings because I got to hold my babies one more time. I didn't want to put them back in their cribs when I was done feeding them. I wanted to just snuggle them a little bit longer. I loved taking them on errands with me because they were my little buddies. I loved finding fun outings for us like the pool, playground, berry farm, and the mall playground. Of course, it was a challenge, having them so close in age, but I loved the challenge. It was what I was made for. Many people get overwhelmed when they have too much on their plate but I thrive on it. It's stimulating and exciting to me. That's why when my life was taken out from under me and I couldn't be the busy bee that I was used to, it was 10 times harder.

In 2009, I was about to have surgery on my gums. Not flattering, I know. Evidently, my overcrowded big honkin' teeth were turned slightly inward, putting pressure on my roots, which had caused some recession. So, I was scheduled to have gum grafts (yuck!). The doctor, Dr. James Culberson in Fredericksburg, Va., assured me this would be a routine procedure and thus I assumed we would get on with life shortly after. You'll find out, this was not the case. I thought, GREAT. We'll get this surgery over lickity split and have our fifth kid that I longed for and pictured.

This surgery was divided into THREE surgeries; top, bottom, and front. For each surgery, I was on a round of antibiotics, an oral steroid pack, anti-inflammatory and pain medication. Holy moly. Little did I know that was nothing compared to all the meds doctors would put me on in the years to come.

Immediately before the surgery I began to have what I thought was a sinus headache. After all, that's all I knew. Looking back, and discussing with doctors, we think I may have experienced migraines as a child but was misdiagnosed. So, I went to my allergy doctor, Dr. Mark Wenger of Allergy Associates of Fredericksburg. He gave me a steroid shot and a Z-pack to get me through the surgery.

I had my first gum graft on Feb. 4, 2009 at Fredericksburg Periodontics and Implant Services. I walked into the office thinking we will get this over with, it may be a hard recovery but I'm tough. I can handle this. I had opted out of anesthesia but I had brought my MP3 player to keep me occupied. Matt had downloaded lots of Nancy Leigh DeMoss talks on there for me. Although Dr. Culberson was a periodontist, the office looked like a typical dental office. On the outside it looked like a little house planted right on Rte. 3. I remember the receptionists not being helpful at all. I lied in the chair more tense than I had ever been in my life. The surgery took several hours and the assistant was resting her entire heavy arm on my bottom jaw. I tried to adjust myself but it was no use. I prayed for every single person I knew during those long hours and thanked God for that time of prayer. I'll get through this, I told myself. I tried to focus hard on the Nancy Leigh DeMoss talks. It helped a little but I couldn't stop thinking about what stage of the surgery they were in and what they were doing with all those instruments in my mouth. Finally, they were done. My mouth was stuffed with this wax-like stuff over where they had operated and gauze. My cheeks were already swollen. Not a pretty picture. Matt had stayed with the kids, so my mom had given me a ride. Home we went. I was anxious about the healing process and about how I would eat. I had battled an eating disorder since college and had already started restricting prior to the surgery. I knew I could only eat soft foods for weeks following and nothing that would crumble and thus possibly get stuck in places that would, let's just say, cause problems. Yuck!

The week following, I had bouts of nausea and a series of night sweats. On February 22, I had an extremely heavy menstrual cycle, so heavy that my OB/GYN, Dr. Kil, also in Fredericksburg, considered it borderline hemorrhaging and put me on 10 days of progesterone.

Leading up to my next gum surgery I continued to have headaches. Still thinking it was the worst sinus headache of my life, I went back to my allergy doctor and he wrote me a prescription for an antibiotic called Biaxin, which had anti-inflammatory properties in it, and gave me another steroid shot. This helped the headaches until the next surgery.

On April 7, 2009, I had my second gum surgery. Going into this, I thought this would be the final surgery. I actually didn't know that there would be a third until leaving that day when I was all swollen and drugged up again. I was devastated and sick to my stomach. My sister drove me this time and I rode home on the brink of throwing up. I barely made it through this surgery and didn't think I could make it through another. Evidently, they do the top, bottom, and then a third surgery for the bottom front. Still, I was tough and mentally I geared up for getting through. My body ached from the tension and anxiety and I walked around with ice packs on my neck for a few days.

This second surgery turned the headaches into a nightmare. They became daily and unbearable. I went to my primary care doctor, Dr. Sampson in Fredericksburg, and part of Mary Washington Healthcare, at the time. (I have since switched to Dr. Dana Brown, of Rappahannock Family Physicians, whom I love.) I entered her office hopeful and thinking it would be a quick fix. I mean, we live in America for goodness sakes! Dr. Sampson thought the headaches were hormonal migraines related to my monthly cycle and gave me a migraine medication called Treximet to try. It worked the first time and then the headaches came back and it wouldn't work anymore. I went back to her office perplexed and she gave me two more migraine medications, Relpax and Imitrex, to try, neither of which helped. Dr. Sampson ordered an MRI (magnetic resonance imaging), which was normal and my allergy doctor ordered a CT (computed tomography) of my sinuses, which also came back normal with the exception of a small bone mass. This bone mass caused the doctors to send me on a "doctor tour" of specialists to make sure it wasn't anything to worry about. For those of you who are dealing with chronic pain and/or fatigue, you know that this is exhausting and feels like "one more thing" to deal with. (I'd learn later that with migraines you can feel sinus pressure because the blood vessels in the lining of the sinus cavity swell). Dr. Smith, another allergy doctor at Allergy Partners of Fredericksburg, put me on a preventative migraine medication called Amitriptyline and Dr. Sampson took me off a few days later.

In April 2009 I saw my neurologist, Dr. Aguilera, at Neurology Associates of Fredericksburg,whom I still see today. I remember having hope that he knew the answer. I thought, "We'll follow his plan and this will all be over and THEN we can have number five." I was still longing for one more baby in all of this. I am sure some of you can't relate to that. Some of you will think having four is a lot. But I'm sure some of you out there know that longing as a mom that seems like it's never going to go away. Thankfully, eventually it did, but not at this point.

Dr. Aguilera diagnosed me with chronic daily migraines and put me on Relafen and Topamax for six months. It seems so general but I was so desperate for an answer that I wanted to believe it. I remember driving home from his office thinking, "We've got this. I've just got to ride this out for six months." Unfortunately, there was no improvement. However, shortly after he did give me the contact information for a doctor in Richmond, Va., Dr. Metzger, who helped me temporarily and eventually directed me to Dr. Marmura at the Jefferson Headache Clinic in Philadelphia, Pa. But we were nowhere close to that yet. Dr. Aguilera would end up sticking it out with me for years.

Shortly after, I took the name and number of a massage therapist in town. I had never had a massage before and she dug deep. I had no idea that a massage wasn't supposed to hurt. My whole body tensed. There was one time that she hit a spot on my shoulder and it radiated through my head just like some of my headaches. Was she on to something? I didn't know. That night I woke up in the middle of the night feeling like I had the flu. For the next few days my whole body ached. As I got ready for a combo birthday party for the kids, I walked around with more ice packs on my head, neck, and shoulders and felt sick and achy. It wasn't until later that I learned that you can feel like this after a massage if your body is trying to rid itself of toxins.

On May 29, 2009, I had my final gum surgery. The headaches were still unbearable and I was beginning to have some jaw pain. I was on a roller coaster of emotions. On one hand, I was determined and focused on getting better. I am an extremely persistent person and I get things done. I saw this as a task at hand and I wasn't going to let anything get in my way. On the other hand, I was grieving over the loss -- the loss of the person that I was, the mom and wife that I was and that I could no longer be with all this pain, and the realization that I was probably not going to have number five. Don't get me wrong. I was SO grateful for the four kids I had. I was SO thankful that God gave me four sweet precious children BEFORE I got sick. But overall, I was simply angry. I was angry because this was not the life that I wanted. What was God doing? How was this good?

I started having itching all over, ear pain, jaw pain, and constant drainage and a sore throat. In May, I also started seeing a chiropractor in town, Dr. Henzler, at Downtown Chiropractic in Fredericksburg, VA, and a massage therapist in his office. I remember having a long conversation with a friend about how much she had been helped by his care and how beneficial chiropractic is to the body. I called his office, and made an appointment right away. I was SO hopeful that this was the answer. I longed that this would take away these blasted headaches. His office wasn't too far from our home. I drove into downtown Fredericksburg to an old quaint home made into an office building. I sat in my yoga pants and V-neck T-shirt waiting for him to come in so I could explain to him my story and eagerly wait for him to say he could make it all better. He didn't seem to be fazed by what I had been through and said I probably had some TMJ left over from the gum surgeries. He recommended that I come in about two times a week for a few weeks and see what he could do. Yes sir! Let's do this. A few weeks passed and I was still gritting my teeth with these darn headaches. The pressure! Why? Dr. Henzler recommended massage. I was scared. I remembered my last massage. He told me that he would talk to the massage therapist and she would be gentle and work up to what I needed. I obliged and keep up with Dr. Henzler's office to this day. Although it didn't get rid of the headaches, I learned the benefits of massage to the body and I firmly believe in continuous self-care through both massage and chiropractic.

People always ask me how I managed. When I look back, I think I have no idea. The kids were so little and I was dealing with an explosive headache every day. But when I was in the midst of it I knew that my kids needed me. I knew I had to get up every morning and provide for their physical needs whether I had a headache or not. When you are a mom, you do what you have to do. I also never wanted to miss out. I loved being a mom. I had always dreamed of being a mom, and this was not going to take that away from me! Noise was hard for me to bear. I would try to keep the noise level down and when Matt called to check in I would ask him to talk as quietly as he could.

Around the same time I began chiropractic, I started seeing a PT at Premier PT down Rte. 3 West in Fredericksburg. This was also my first time seeing a physical therapist. I walked into the office and they paired me up with a therapist. She listened to my story and recommended dry needling. Dry needling is when they stick needles into trigger points. The idea is that the trigger point tightens and then releases. I knew enough to know that I was tight and most likely had a lot of trigger points. The therapist did dry needling mostly in my head. I went back several times a week and the therapist also used electrical stim. I didn't notice anything with the dry needling but the electrical stim made the pain get 100 times worse. I remember being home with the kids and calling Matt at work crying asking him to come home. I am not an easy crier. I never cry. So, he knew it was bad. This is not to say anything against PT. It just evidently was not the right treatment for me at the time. Keep in mind, this was a long journey with a lot going on.

In June 2009, I started having itching all over. It became severe and I couldn't sleep at night. The ear and jaw pain got more constant. I had pins and needles all over from the Topamax. I began to have horrible sinus and nasal congestion. I felt sickly all the time and felt like I had the flu. I was barely getting around the house. I began to notice that I was sensitive to chemicals and fragrances. I remember being in Target and walking down the detergent aisle. It was like a wave of something came over me from head to toe. I felt it in my head, neck, and then whole body. I got violently ill and was in immediate pain. I started sneezing over and over and walked as fast as I could out of the store leaving my cart behind. I sat in the car hoping it would pass. I drove home and went to bed. What had happened to me? I couldn't tolerate being around things that I used to. I was having food intolerances and sensitivities. I was having abdominal pain and bloating from foods that I used to be able to eat. In July, I began to have horrible neck, shoulder, ear and jaw pain in addition to sharp pains darting through my face. What was happening to me? I felt like I was falling apart. I didn't like feeling out of control.

I saw an ear nose and throat doctor, Dr. Dash, at the Ear Nose and Throat and Facial Plastic Surgery Center in Fredericksburg, who said the ear and jaw pain would settle down. When!? Why don't these doctors have answers?

Soon after, labs showed that my liver enzymes were slightly elevated. This could explain the itching. The jaw and ear pain continued. I tried some new supplements from a friend out of desperation. She knew a lot about nutrition and I needed help. My neck continued to feel like it was on fire and my head continued to feel like it was about to explode. So much pressure. So much pain.

In September, I finally got in with Dr. Metzger in Richmond, Va., who was an oral and facial surgeon recommended by Dr. Aguilera, my Fredericksburg neurologist at Neurology Associates of Fredericksburg. This was a long drive down to Richmond. But I would do anything that might help move me in the right direction. I walked into his office and checked in. I sat down in the waiting room longing to just feel normal again. When I got called back, I was shown to a room that looked like a typical dental office room with the dental chair that reclines. He took some X-rays and said the disc in my jaw had been dislocated during the gum surgery and all I needed was a muscle relaxant. After two muscle relaxants failed, he gave me Valium and I had no headaches for three weeks! Cured! It was heaven! I loved Valium! Then they started coming back and I was nauseated and fatigued. I remember the first headache that came back after three headache-free weeks. I bolted up in my bed both shocked and frightened. No, this can't be. Are you kidding me? I felt defeated. I can't keep doing this. The neck pain began to get worse as well so Dr. Metzger added Feldene for eight months with the Valium.

In November 2009, I was still battling the headaches and fatigue and began to have bouts of severe abdominal pain. I had had abdominal pain before but this had me doubled over in pain for most of the day. My husband ended up taking me to the ER. Thankfully, my dad and stepmom drove over to take care of the kids. After hours, they found nothing and it eventually subsided. These bouts continued and my primary care doctor put me on Prevacid for eight weeks. No improvement. She sent me to a urologist, GI doctor and OB/GYN. Seeing these specialists, of course they began tests galore, including scopes in and out of everywhere, X-rays, an endoscopy, colonoscopy, ultrasound of my gall bladder, more MRIs, CT scans, blood work, etc. We made several more trips to the ER. The pain stopped me in my tracks. No answers. More tests. The bouts were getting longer. Up to three hours of intense pain. More procedures. They sent me to follow up with a urologist in town. I was overwhelmed. I couldn't be sick. I had to take care of my kids! Moms can't be sick.

I remember getting the call. After all these tests, the urologist found that my left kidney was swollen and there was a narrowing at the ureteropelvic junction (UPJ). I remember crying and falling into Matt's arms and saying, "I don't want one more thing to be wrong with me." Why was all this happening? Why was my body betraying me? Wasn't I just healthy and strong the other day? Where did that body go?

Karis and Connor would never remember me being healthy and strong. I grieved. I wanted my other life back. I wanted the life that I wanted. I tried to pray but I was angry. I remember thinking at one point, "I'll get better with or without you, God." That's how bad it was.

I remember walking in the neighborhood, on one of my "good" days, yelling at God, and yet preaching to myself that He is good, His plan was best and that He loved me. I remember telling my kids that over and over, that even though Mommy was sick, God's plan was best. I never wanted them to doubt God's goodness, but I was struggling.

I felt like a failure as a mom. I was still homeschooling my kids and my kids' learning was suffering. I worried about them. Should we put them in public school? Should we put them in private school? There were days that I'd start school and I'd have to stop, put a movie on for the kids, and go to sleep. I remember one day that I was in tears because the medication I was on was making me so tired and I couldn't sleep. We ended up getting involved in co-ops to fill the gaps but that was exhausting for me and sometimes I had to leave early to go home and take a nap. There were times I'd sit in co-op in a daze.

God knew everything that was happening to me. He wasn't surprised. He wasn't throwing His hands in the air saying, "Oh, crap, I can't believe all of this is happening to Ariel! What am I going to do!?" No, He knew and even when it seemed as if God wasn't there or like He wasn't working or answering prayers He was.

I had to keep speaking the Truth to myself and trusting Him. I knew that God doesn't waste our pain.

I saw another chiropractor in town who told me to start doing detox baths with apple cider vinegar or aluminum-free baking soda with the water as hot as I could stand it to sweat out toxins. I continued this for several months.

I had lots of visits with several urologists. I also got lots of opinions and lots of medications.

In December 2009, we decided to go with Dr. Berry, a urologist in Fredericksburg who would do the surgery on my UPJ robotically. This would be the least invasive. For the meantime, he wanted to put in a stent. This was done in the hospital. The room was FREEZING and doctors surrounded me. I was awake but couldn't see anything that was happening because of a sheet that separated my upper half from the lower. I remember a nurse throwing blankets on me to help me stay warm. I just wanted it to be over. The stent was supposed to help with nausea and abdominal pain. Surprise, it didn't. When I got home I had this weird headache. It wasn't like my normal headaches. It felt like a "dry" headache, I kept telling Matt. Then it clicked. The anesthesiologist had warned us about this. The spinal didn't heal properly, which caused additional headaches and a trip to the ER to get a patch.

In January 2010, I had the recommended surgery to fix my UPJ. Although this was done robotically it was still a five-day stay in the hospital for recovery and six-week recovery at home. My body took longer than normal to wake up from the anesthesia and this meant extra X-rays every day to see where my organs were as far as waking up. Dr. Berry took off my ureter and reattached it where it should be at the bottom and cut out a narrow portion of it. Surprisingly, I had no abdominal pain or nausea for six weeks post op. I went for my follow up for him to remove the stent that was put in post op thinking that this, this had finally fixed part of the puzzle. At least the abdominal pain and nausea were gone! I still had the fatigue and headaches but at least we were getting somewhere! At least we had some answers! When he removed the stent, all the pain came back, along with the nausea. I fell on my knees beside my bed and gave everything I could over to the Lord. But really, I didn't want this. This is not what I pictured for my life. Could this really be Your best, God?

Dr. Berry ordered an ultrasound, IVP (intravenous pyelogram) test, and renal scan and couldn't find anything. Everything looked great on paper! I got passed around to a few doctors who ordered a whole other array of tests with no answers. This was exhausting while dealing with daily headaches, nausea, abdominal pain, and chronic fatigue. Dr. Berry put me on Pyridium in case I was having bladder spasms. No help. I was getting weary and sick of medications and tests.

I was frustrated with conventional doctors. They seemed to be focusing on the symptoms instead of the underlying cause. I decided to see a functional medicine doctor in the area, Dr. Anderson, in Fredericksburg. He had me do the LEAP (Lifestyle Eating and Performance) food allergy test and a stool test. It showed I had some food sensitivities, low immune system, malabsorption issues, and compromised gut. He put me on a few supplements but after a while of that, I wasn't really satisfied. I still felt awful every single day. My body dragged. My head felt like it was going to explode. I never knew when the next abdominal attack would hit. I often wanted to just lie in bed all day with the covers over my head and sleep until this was all over. I felt this tug of war between wanting to take care of my kids, enjoy every second of their lives and my body not being able to keep up with that. My body needed more.

As I was searching for answers, I started seeing a (Nambudripad's Allergy Elimination Techniques) NAET practitioner in March 2010 in Richmond VA. At this point I had not gotten anywhere with conventional doctors. I had been through the ringer of tests and meds with no help. Don't get me wrong. I am thankful for them and thankful to be in America where we can get the medical help we need and get it quickly. But I wasn't getting what I needed at this point, so I began to search elsewhere. I pulled up to the office and walked through the winding hallway to find her suite. She had a tiny little office painted green and it was divided by a curtain. When I entered there was a desk and chair where we talked about what I was going through and what the treatment would be like. Then we went behind the curtain. There was a table where I would lie and be "cleared" of the substances that I was reacting to. I continued seeing the NAET practitioner through July before quitting. I wasn't getting anywhere and it was expensive and over an hour away. I also saw two acupuncturists; one in Richmond and one in Fredericksburg. It was slow going but I stuck it out for months with each of them. Again, it was expensive considering insurance doesn't cover it, and I was going several times a week on top of everything else.

Seeing the NAET practitioner was an experience. She had boxes and boxes of vials containing the "energy" to different objects or substances. It could be food, environmental things; you name it, she had it. Then she muscle-tested me to see where my body was most sensitive, and we would "clear" my body. To clear me she would push on acupressure points on my back and then I would have to avoid that substance for 24 hours. I ended up seeing another NAET practitioner down the road in Fredericksburg, who did things a little differently but it's the same idea of working with energy. The second NAET practitioner I saw used a computer and device to test me, as opposed to muscle testing and then cleared me with actual acupuncture needles. I just wanted to get better. I didn't care how. I was willing to try anything and I knew people who had actually gotten better through NAET. I'm not knocking anything!

Chapter 3: More Symptoms

It was a spiral downward in April 2010. The fatigue was worse and constant. Have you ever felt like you are trying to stay awake while taking sleeping pills? Yeah. I began to have brain fog, body aches, hair loss, tight and sore muscles, flu-l ke symptoms, abdominal spasms, digestive issues, cramping, and pelvic pain.

I don't know what was worse -- the symptoms or the stress of trying to get better and worrying about the kids. When you are a mom, being ill not only affects you, it affects the entire family. I felt responsible and guilty. I felt alone. But, as a mom, I have kids. I have to keep going. I had to get up every mornirg. And THANK YOU, GOD, for those rays of sunshine! I had so many reasons to be grateful, so I kept moving through the motions of every day. I wanted to make sure my kids had everything they needed and that their lives went on without interruption.

In June 2010, my gut was a mess. I was bloated, in pain and nauseous all the time. I remember going to my GI doctor, Dr. Lee at Gastroenterology Associates of Fredericksburg, and being exhausted from sitting in one more doctor's office. Dr. Lee gave me Bentyl to help stop what he thought were spasms and, Dr. Brown, my primary care doctor, gave me Amitiza to help with the constipation and bloating. The Amitiza gave me shortness of breath and chest pain. The Bentyl made me more constipated, eye roll. I was feeling so sick and run down. I'd walk through the house in a daze and sometimes just collapse wherever I was. I lived most of my life on the couch or the bed and let the kids play around me. I came down with a bad case of eczema and athlete's foot for the first time in my life, and came down with strep all at once. Clearly, my immune system was suffering. Also at this time my primary care doctor ordered an ultrasounc of my pelvis because of all the spasms. It showed one small cyst. I was extremely exhausted from all the tests and from dealing with all my symptoms. I was exasperated and hopeless from nothing working. I decided it was time to do something more radical. So, I weaned off all of my medications and decided to once again seek out a more alternative route. Keep in mind I was still having daily headaches.

This was when I started seeing a new NAET practitioner. This time, closer to home, in Fredericksburg.This practitioner had me bring everything from my house one batch at a time to "clear" me from the actual things that I was coming in contact with every day. Her office was up several flights of stairs. I would trudge up the stairs carrying as many heavy items and bags of goods as I possibly could with my weak body week after week. Unfortunately, I still did not see improvement after going through her full protocol through December 2010. She had me do a test that came back positive for E. coli, so I was treated for that by a doctor. Unfortunately even after being cleared from that, I didn't feel any better.

In July 2010, I began to see a compounding pharmacist at South River Pharmacy in Richmond. He worked closely with an OB/GYN, Dr. Miller also in Richmond, who practiced functional medicine. This was my first more in-depth experience with a functional medicine doctor. I walked into the pharmacy to a little office in the back. I told him my story, longing for him to say that he could help. He listened and recommended a lot of tests. Then he took me out into the store and placed a good number of supplements into a basket. I was up for anything at this point. Just give me whatever will make me feel better.

The labs I had to get through Dr. Miller: These tests were to check   hormones, thyroid, iron, Lyme disease, bacteria, parasites, yeast, malabsorption, gluten sensitivity, heavy metal toxicity, and more. Some of this was blood work, some urine, and I also gave a hair sample. My progesterone and testosterone were extremely low, as well as my iron, vitamin D, and B12. My reverse T3 was abnormal. I had a severe gluten intolerance as well as major malabsorption issues and a buildup of toxins. I tested negative for Lyme; however, if you know anything about Lyme tests this is incredibly debatable and I would test positive several times in the near future. When I left the store, in addition to the supplements and vitamins, I also left with hormonal replacements, a detox shake, and B12 shots.

From August through December 2010, I began to see a PT in northern Virginia to help with the pelvic floor pain. Her name was Cora at a cute little office at Women's Health PT. This was recommended by a friend who had gotten significant help from this particular therapist. Cora massaged my pelvic muscles as well as used an ultrasound on the pelvic muscles. I continued the supplements from Dr. Miller and continued appointments with him, as well as his supplements and medications.

At this time, I also noticed I could no longer go into stores without getting a migraine and what seemed to be an allergic reaction. My incident in Target was the first of many. Any sort of chemical, perfume, laundry detergent, cleaner, etc., would do the same thing. We went fragrance free in our entire house and I avoided smells like the plague. Even when I gave someone a hug or brushed by someone who was wearing perfume, lotion, or had a fragrant detergent, it would trigger a reaction that could last days or weeks. I felt like I had to live in a bubble. I wanted my life back.

We replaced all of the harmful chemical cleaners in our home with Norwex. Around this same time, I started learning about the dangers of our personal hygiene products. I begin reading labels like you wouldn't believe. I threw out our shampoos, our deodorant, my makeup, our soap. You get the idea. My body needed all the help it could get and I wanted my kids to grow up in a safe environment. Some of the products I now use are Kiss My Face olive oil bar soap, Norwex cleaning products, John Master's Fragrance Free Shampoo and Conditioner, Derma E Facial Cleanser, Jane Iredale MakeUp, and Schmidt's Fragrance Free Deodorant Stick.

During this time my nose was burning, my eyes were watering and itching, I started having muscle twitches all over my body, my blood pressure was very low and I continued to be extremely tired. I struggled with moodiness, anxiety, and depression during the last few months of the summer. In November, I started looking at nutrition and began a grain/dairy/starch/sugar- free diet and began the GAPS diet for gut healing. This diet eliminates a lot of foods and has several stages. The goal and idea was good but, unfortunately, this caused me to lose a lot of weight and I didn't have weight to lose.

I remember researching the hyperbaric oxygen chambers but they were only available in California and Florida at the time and I would have had to live there for three months away from my kids without guarantee that they would work. Should I take that chance, with the expense? It wasn't covered by insurance. We looked into the Hansa center in the Midwest. I knew someone that it had helped. Again, they didn't take insurance. I would go out there and live for at least six weeks and it would cost a good $20K when we added up all the expenses and the possible second trip out there. And what if it didn't help? Sometimes things just seemed hopeless. But I knew I had to keep pressing on. I had to find answers. My kids were my driving force.

At times my fatigue was so severe that I couldn't even walk up the stairs in my own house. No matter how much I slept, it was never enough. The migraines were unbearable and I was having night sweats. Simple things like sweeping the floor seemed like monumental tasks.

In December, I stopped PT when the pelvic floor muscles became tighter despite treatment. The therapist said it was due to stress. Go figure. At this time, I also went back to Dr. Anderson's office to see the PA. She suggested we clean up our home -- air ducts cleaned, allergen covers, air purifiers, etc. We did. I did not notice any improvement but I'm sure they were good things to do. She also had me reduce my diet down to meat, veggies, poultry, and fish. I still felt awful. She gave me shots of magnesium, B6, and calcium for a while, along with supplements of olive leaf and several homeopathics. I felt overwhelmed with the money we were spending and I was not feeling better. Despite everything we were trying I was still battling the headaches, fatigue, abdominal pain and flulike symptoms.

I heard about ionic foot baths and found someone in the area who did them, so I made an appointment. I walked up to the little house called The Natropath in Fredericksburg. It was an old little house on Lafayette Boulevard bursting with supplements and natural treatments. The man behind the counter took me into a back room and got me set up. I slid my bare feet into the basin filled with water and a metal device and watched the water turn to different colors and eventually brown with foam on top, which is said to be because of yeast. After 30 minutes my session was complete and the person helping me gave me electrolytes for me to drink. Did it help? I don't know.

I was exhausted from going to doctors without any real answers. Didn't America have the best doctors in the world? Why weren't we getting anywhere? I knew something was really wrong with me. I used to like going out and being social but I was losing my enjoyment in life. I struggled to even enjoy the little things much less anything else. The brain fog was thick and it was hard to think of words like I used to be able to. I used to be a great communicator and now I struggled to get out full sentences. The thoughts were there but I couldn't get them out to make complete sense.

Out of desperation I started doing some more reading on nutrition. I started really digging on my own. This is something I had control over. This is something I didn't have to depend on doctors for. I slowly began to learn by reading online. I ordered some books...I started making some small changes.

I tried to stay hopeful. But I was frustrated and worried. I had such a decline in my health with no real answers. The doctors seemed to have an excuse for every symptom but nothing actually seemed to get better.

In March 2011, I found Dr. Zackrison at Optimal Health Dimensions in Fairfax, Va. I was going to a weekly Bible Study and a lady there heard that I was suffering with chronic pain among other things. She introduced me to another lady at the same Bible Study who had gone to Dr. Z and had been helped. Thank you, Lord, for putting me and these two ladies in the same paths! Dr. Z is a rheumatologist by trade but also specialized in Lyme disease and other autoimmune diseases. I had to see Wendy, her NP, first because that is the way her office works. I LOVE Wendy. Suspecting Lyme, she started me on Doxycycline right away. She listened to my story and began treating me one to two times a week immediately with IVs that were homeopathic and anti-bacterial/viral/fungal. They also contained minerals and vitamins that my body desperately needed along with pushes of glutathione. In my excitement that I had finally found help, I told my mother about Dr. Z and she criticized me and told me that she was just taking my money. That was so far from the truth. In fact, Dr. Z was not only gracious in her physical care for me but also very gracious and kind financially. Dr. Z always searches for the newest treatments for her patients and never settles. This is typical for Lyme patients, to not have the support of their family and friends because it is so controversial. Please, persevere! I wish you all the blessings in your health journey! You CAN do it and you CAN get better!

When I finally got to see Dr. Z, I could tell she wasn't messing around. She knew her stuff and she knew me better than

I knew myself. I loved that she was an MD but also was very alternative, so that she could pull from both sides. The atmosphere was warm and friendly. Her staff was so helpful and caring. My first time back to the IV room I was overwhelmed with gratitude for the amount of people she was helping and my heart was heavy with how many people were hurting, as there were at least 10 chairs lined up in a row with people in pain with IVs dripping. In addition, there were chairs along the side wall with people waiting for their IVs. What would we do without Dr. Z? As I sat in the IV chair myself I saw an entire family that was infected with Lyme. My heart ached for them as they struggled to get healthy. I met a woman whose marriage had fallen apart because she was putting everything she had into getting better. I met a woman whose brother was driving her to and from every appointment because she was too sick to take herself. My heart swelled with admiration for the love they had for each other and how they stuck together, side by side, as she sought out treatment. And I met new friends, friends that I would text and support and they would support me. Friends that we shared our new protocols and encouraged each other to press on when it got tough and seemed hopeless. We became a community and a family. We were the ones that understood each other and would stand by each other till the end.

Dr. Z used a device called the ASYRA (tests and works with your energy), as well as blood tests that showed Lyme disease and co-infections. I wracked my brain and thought back to when I was younger. I know I had gotten bitten by multiple ticks from wandering in my grandparents' woods. But I didn't know the danger of them. My mom just plucked them off with tweezers. I had never noticed a bull's-eye but I was also never looking for that. Because I'd carried this for a long time I would need many rounds of treatment and multiple sets of antibiotics. It's important to note here that the ELISA test and Western Blot test are the typical tests used for testing Lyme disease. When I was tested I did have several bands show up. However, the ELISA and WB aren't always sensitive enough to pick up on chronic Lyme. The lab compares your band pattern to what the Centers for Disease Control has considered characteristic of the one found with Lyme. According to the CDC you need five of the ten bands for a Lyme diagnosis. However, some of the bands are more significant than others. So, if you have one of these bands without the others you could still have Lyme. Another issue is that not all the labs use the same means to analyze the Western Blot, so you can get a positive result if your blood is sent to one lab and a negative one if your blood is sent to another. You must work with a Lyme specialist if you have chronic Lyme in order to get a proper diagnosis! Unfortunately, 56% of people get a negative test when they actually do have Lyme. According to the VA Board of Physicians and most conventional doctors, the standard treatment for Lyme is 28 days of antibiotics. Three weeks of antibiotics will not cure chronic Lyme Disease. So many people continue to suffer.

Dr. Z continued the Doxycycline and added Ceftin, both antibiotics, for the Lyme and co-infections. She put me on adrenal and thyroid support, which I desperately needed, as well as a combination hormone cream. She also treated me for parasites and yeast.

I was continuing IV treatment several times a week. My veins are naturally small and tend to roll and blow but after months and months of IVs and blood work they were scarred as well, so it was very difficult for the nurses to find a good vein. It was not unusual for them to stick me multiple times. They would put heat on my arms and hands to help. There was one time I got stuck 17 times before they got a good vein. I didn't mind, though. I knew I needed my treatment. Blood work was easier because they could use a small needle, but for the IV treatments they needed a good vein that would hold up. Dr. Z has a strict policy that the nurses only stick the patient two times. The times that the nurses stuck me more than twice was with my blessing as I desperately wanted my treatment.

My sister's wedding was coming up and if you have ever dealt with a chronic illness you know that any kind of event like this is terrifying. Questions were racing through my mind like, "How will I get through? Will I be able to enjoy any of it?" Just thinking about the logistics was exhausting. Then the anger set in. "Why can't I just enjoy my sister's wedding? Why am I STILL dealing with this pain and fatigue and these doctors and why can't they figure it out? Why am I so tired, and why can't I just enjoy life for crying out loud!? Why, why, why?"

It was so easy to fall into a pity party. Why couldn't I be the mom that I wanted to be!? I remember thinking, "Is this REALLY Your best, God? REALLY? Because my plan looks a whole lot better! Look at these precious kids you gave me and I can't even take care of them! I can't even enjoy them God! You gave me this amazing life and I can't even enjoy it! I don't understand God! Please!?"

One thing through all of this is that I tried REALLY HARD to be a good mom. I never wanted my kids to look back and think they missed out on anything "because mom was sick." I pushed the pain and fatigue aside and looked for fun things to do with them like every mom does. I still wanted to do the "mom things" like taking them to their activities. I wanted to be the mom and I wanted them to be able to pursue THEIR dreams. I never wanted to hold them back because they had a sick mom. I tried really hard and it was exhausting.

It was now spring 2011 and my weight had dropped significantly. I added back in some food to gain weight for the wedding and my body did NOT like it. I had been on a very strict diet of gluten free, dairy free and sugar free. When I introduced these foods back into my diet, I had bloating beyond belief. I was SO miserable it brought me to tears. It took months for my body to recover. But, hey, I gained weight for the wedding. I realized that my diet was a huge part of what was going on with me, so I quickly reverted to my strict diet after the wedding.

Chapter 4: The Power of Plants

I continued to research nutrition and learned that plants are powerful. Everything came back to plants. I started devouring books on healthy living regarding diet. I radically changed mine, mainly because I was desperate. After a few months, Matt jumped on board with me.

The one thing that everything I read had in common was that plants were powerful. I bought a dehydrator, a juicer, and a Vitamix. I started chopping, mixing, juicing, and tried to get as many plants into my body and into my kids' bodies as possible. I always felt like I fell short because I knew more was better! The juicer and dehydrator were always a mess and I was exhausted. Not to mention picky eaters! We also put in a reverse osmosis water filter under our sink. We put water filters on all the tubs and showers. So much is absorbed through our skin and I wanted to be careful. I had a lot of fear. I wanted to do everything right both for me and my family.

I kept reading about the benefits of plants and all the good things they did in the body. I felt like we could never get enough. All the prep was exhausting, not to mention the food quality today was frustrating to say the least. I learned that I had to eat way more quantity to get the same amount of nutrients than our ancestors did only 50 years ago. We were also spending loads of money on organic produce because my body needed the cleanest possible and I certainly didn't want to give my kids any less.

I also read on Dr. Mercola's website that there are plants that clean the air. So I bought plants for the house. I was doing everything I could for my health. Everything. I had always been a persistent person, a hard worker, someone who never gave up. This was no different. I wasn't only doing it for me. I wanted to get better for my family. This affected my husband and my kids. I wanted to get better for them!

I read a lot about EFT (tapping or Emotional Freedom Technique). I found a practitioner who specialized in it in Northern VA. His name was Kevin. I saw him once in person and did some therapy over skype. I watched some webinars on it and read some more. Some very respected doctors believe in it. I started to learn more about the body and energy pathways. It fascinated me but I really got nowhere with tapping as far as actually feeling any difference.

I read about grounding and the miracles that people were experiencing. Since I'm not going to lie around in the dirt I bought Dr. Mercola's grounding mat. I slept on it every night for years.

In August 2011, not only did I begin seeing a dietician, Kelley Reatzech and Laura Powell FNP, but we also flew to Arizona to see an ND, Daniel Smith, that a friend of ours recommended. She had a whole array of health issues and he was able to get her stable again. Matt and hopped on a plane to Arizona to see this Daniel Smith because what did have we to lose? We had tried too much and here we were hearing of a friend that had been healed by leaps and bounds by this Daniel. We would never know if we didn't try. We drove into this little almost deserted town to find his office. He used muscle testing and gave me a protocol for Lyme, including high doses of HCL and iodine for three months. He also found a low-grade infection in my upper gums that he wanted to treat with neem oil and super nano green tea for radiation detox. I didn't notice anything significant from his treatment but we tried.

Additionally, at this time I was getting chelation through IV with Dr. Zackrison. This was to break up the biofilms to let out more of the microorganisms (bacteria, parasites, fungi, for example) that we needed to kill. Our body is amazing. It protects itself by creating biofilms that collect harmful things in our bodies.

66

It's very hard to break up these biofilms but in order to rea ly get my body cleaned out we needed to break them up and get the "bugs" out, as Dr. Z called them. With most bacter a, when given antibiotics, they die. However, with chronic Lyme, they create biofilm around themselves that antibiotics cannot penetrate. So you have to break up the biofilms to let out the Lyme bacteria and then attack them with antibiotics. This is very hars¬ on the body, so you have to support the immune system at the same time as well as detox. I also started coffee enemas to help detoxify the liver.

Dr. Z added Alinia and Praziquantel, both anti parasite drugs, as well as Cipro (an antibiotic) to my medications, so that as the microorganisms in the biofilms were released, my body would be protected. Once the biofilms have been broken up and the Lyme is in your bloodstream you can test positive on the ELISA and Western Blot even if you tested negative previously. It's also important to note that the ELISA test only picks up 50-65 % of Lyme cases. You can also get a negative result if you were infected with a strain of Lyme or co-infections that the CDC approved Lyme tests can't detect. There are more than 100 strains of Lyme in the U.S. and more than 300 strains worldwide. The test doesn't test for all of these strains. So, if you have some of the strains that the tests aren't looking for you could have a negative result but still have Lyme. This is why it is so important to find a Lyme specialist to work with, so that he or she can diagnose you early by your symptoms.

Dr. Z also adjusted my thyroid medication. I also started some stem cell shots with Dr. Z through October 2011. Thankfully, some of my hormones came back to normal during this time.

Dr. Z eventually asked me to do my first liver cleanse. This consists of eating a mainly all-liquid diet throughout the day followed by two glasses of apple juice, olive oil, and salt. It was so hard to get down, I thought I was going to be sick. I went to bed

67

straight after the second glass. The next morning I couldn't get out of bed other than to crawl to the bathroom. Let's just say I was running like a bathtub faucet, over and over and over. I slept all day in between bouts. I didn't see any stones but who knows, it was coming out so fierce and harshly. I never experienced anything like it. I was weaker than I had ever been in my life.

At first Matt was taking off work to watch the kids for my appointments. They were so little when it all started. But when the appointments kept going on and on this was not realistic. I started to ask my mom and my mother-in-law for help. However, I began to feel like my mom didn't understand and like I owed her, so I started taking the kids with me. The kids packed all their school supplies and electronics. It was an ordeal in and of itself to get them all out the door while feeling like I had the flu, but we eventually piled in the van. Whenever we took long trips to a doctor's office we set up a movie in the van. The kids chatted about who got to pick what movie on the way there and on the way back. I thanked God for those videos. We lugged all their school work, snacks, lunches, electronics, and coloring books up the stairs, into the elevator, and down the long hallways into the waiting room. The receptionists and nurses loved seeing my kids and always made them feel right at home. Dr. Z's office had a kids' play area, so the kids set up camp and got busy. They played and played and played during my IV and office visit and always knew where to find me. They took some time out to get some school work done and would squeeze in next to me in the IV chair to ask me school questions and to get some snuggles and hugs. They never forgot to come ask for money for the vending machine. Thankfully, it was full of healthy snacks and green juices, so I always said yes. I dug in my purse and pulled out some money for each of them. They were patient as I finished my IV, had my office visit, still had to get labs done and then went to the supplement store to get my bag of necessary supplements for my new protocol. Then I still had to check out. This was a full day every visit. It was even longer if I had to do the ASSYRA or CESDA. We gathered all our belongings and headed back to the car where the kids put on another movie. As soon as we got home I crawled into bed, as it was an exhausting day for me. The kids would finish their school work and I'd answer more questions later that night. They are such good kids.

Matt's cousin told me about an orthogonal chiropractor, Dr. Lim, at the Spine Arts Center in Springfield, Va., who had helped her with her headaches. Really? I wanted help with my headaches! I began seeing the same orthogonal chiropractor in northern Virginia, about an hour and a half from my home. She works on the axis with a machine. I got some relief from the headaches but it wasn't lasting. I had to travel back and forth so frequently that it was exhausting. The kids liked coming to this doctor with me because she had snacks in the wa ting room. We hooked up a movie on the DVD player in the van and brought their school work with us. I kept it up for about a year. I kept Dr. Z in the loop about the orthogonal chiropractor and Dr. Z started me on Ketek for a tick-borne bacteria around this same time.

Meanwhile, I started getting allergy shots again and continued those for years. Evidently, all my childhood allergies decided to come back. My body is literally screaming from the inside out.

All of the sudden the nausea got extremely intense, combined with racing heart and shortness of breath. Wendy and Dr. Z agreed that it was my gall bladder. She ordered a CT scan and a HIDA (hepatobiliary iminodiacetic acid) scan of my gall bladder. The HIDA is a scan done at the hospital. I had to fast and lie on a table almost like an MRI. I was injected with a contrast through my vein and the table slides into a huge machine while pictures are taken. They both came back normal. However, Bartonella and Babesia, both tick-borne infections, both came back positive on my recent labs. Dr. Z ordered IV antibiotics. I got a peripherally inserted central catheter (PICC)line at Reston Hospital on December 5 and started home care for five months. I was nervous about getting a PICC line as it was very invasive but what was I to do? At this point I felt like I had to trust Dr. Z and I did like that the antibiotic going through the PICC line would bypass the gut, as antibiotics are so hard on the digestive tract. I remember lying on the hospital bed and the nurses asking me some probing questions about why I was getting the PICC line like it was any of their business. For five months, I had to care for the PICC line in my arm. I had to make sure it was tightly covered when I showered. I had to be home for our scheduled home care time so that the home nurse could clean and check it. I had to hook myself up to the IV pole every day for five months and my kids witnessed this. But all in all, it didn't bother me. I was finding my way, my road to recovery. All in all, I am thankful. I am thankful that Dr. Z was hitting everything from every angle. I was too tired to care for myself and she was caring for me. I think that was what was most important to me – that while I was too overwhelmed and too exhausted and sickly to think or care for myself, Dr. Z was thinking and caring for me and hitting this illness from all angles. Everyone who is facing a chronic illness needs a doctor like this!

Dr. Z also increased my thyroid medication, gave me a double dose of the antibacterial Ketek, started me on Reglan to help move my bowels, which had slowed significantly. I remember being so bloated my stomach couldn't stretch anymore. I tried everything from aloe to slippery elm, to the normal things like hydration and fiber and massaging the bowels. No luck. Dr. Z recommended me to start hydrotherapy (the CT scan revealed an almost blockage in the upper right abdomen). That is why my digestive symptoms were so unbearable! Thank you, God, for the CT scan! Hydrotherapy uses water to flush out the lower bowel. More on what this is in the chapter on health coaching. This was a life saver for me! It's incredibly important in Lyme patients to detox through all the main detox pathways.

She increased Nystatin to four times per day to combat the antibiotics. Nystatin kills yeast and fungus that can easily accumulate when on antibiotics. Unfortunately, the Nystatin made me so nauseated I had to stop. She had me begin Actigall as well to help my gallbladder during the antibiotics.

I continued to meet new people in the IV room. Most people I met never saw a bull's-eye rash and none of them got cured with the conventionally recommended three weeks of antibiotics. The longer they went untreated, the more symptoms arose.

We wondered why we had to search all over the US, and sometimes all over the world for treatments and often with no solution or improvement. We wondered why traditional doctors weren't able to diagnose, have a plan, or prescribe proper tools. We wondered why we had encountered doctors along our journey that had told us Lyme wasn't real, didn't exist, or it was all in our heads.

Chapter 5: A Hypnotist? I'll Try Anything!

At this point, in December 2011, I am not doing so well emotionally and Dr. Z recommends a hypnotist. Hmmm...CK. I'll try anything at this point. His name is Dr. Wieslaw Rocki, in Fairfax, Va. Dr. Rocki has me focusing on gratitude and thankfulness in EVERY situation.

My entire attitude and perspective shift. Matt notices a difference and so do the kids. I am able to be happy and peaceful even though my symptoms have not yet changed. Dr. Rocki has me assuming the positive future at all times, and realizing that I cannot control any person or circumstance. Imagine that. I can only control myself, therefore I need to let things go. He also helps me recognize negative thought patterns and cycles to break (control, anger, shame...which only makes things worse.) and replace them with acceptance, unconditional acceptance. This acceptance breaks the control cycle. He also made me realize that I have a lot of anger toward myself and even self-hate for not being able to fix my illness. I've been trying so hard. So hard. I'm tired. Why can't I fix this? Why won't God let me fix this? Why is God standing in my way? Am I still angry at God? I know I'm not supposed to be angry at God. I don't want my kids to know I'm angry at God...so many questions I can't answer.

Karis, my youngest, loved to dance. I loved watching her dance around the living room while I lay on the couch feeling sickly and in pain. Watching her made me happy.

I finally had a positive doctor visit. My most recent labs with Dr. Z showed that everything was improving! All three bacteria went down, autoimmune activity improved, thyroid came up slightly, white count came up, potassium came up, B12 was finally good! Yay! I was having fewer headaches and less fatigue, less nausea, and feeling better emotionally. I had some hope again. Maybe I was turning a corner. Maybe I was getting better! Dr. Z still wanted me to continue hydrotherapy for my gut, try Nystatin again because of the antibiotics I was on, continue a potassium Rx, and all supplements (there are a LOT!). This was the beginning of January 2012.

By the end of January 2012, my weight hit an all-time low, my vitamin A and potassium were so low I had to get a potassium IV and the headaches and fatigue had increased again! Why? It was discouraging to say the least. I tried to stay positive and thankful. Dr. Rocki tried to help me get my weight up. My eating disorder mindset was strong and I was trying to fight it.

In March 2012, I started a new drug, Domperidone, for my bowels, and was eating lots of nutrient dense, high-calorie foods to keep my weight up. Dr. Z increased my thyroid meds and switched my IV antibiotics. This triggered horrible headaches and worsening digestive symptoms. Dr. Z said that meant it was working. Die-off can be strong but necessary. When enormous populations of bacteria are killed off with antibiotics they release endotoxins and biotoxins into the blood and tissues faster than the body can handle. The immune system reacts with a range of awful symptoms, such as chills, muscle stiffness, headaches, muscle and joint pain, fever, flu-like symptoms, basically the same things I was already feeling, so it was hard to tell what was die-off and what were my normal symptoms. So I pressed on.

The appointments with Dr. Z were a roller coaster. I was going to her office twice a week for IVs and seeing her once a month for an office visit. I was still feeling awful, battling the daily headaches, nausea, abdominal pain, and bloating, brain fog, and this overall sickly feeling. So, I came into her office discouraged but by the time I left I was hopeful again. She would have all my labs and have a good solid plan. Her hopefulness was contagious. I could tell she was knowledgeable and experienced. I had seen patients leave her office healthy again. I knew God could get me healthy and I knew she could, too. Just why was it so hard? I'd leave her office with the plan and encouraged only to have another hard month and come back discouraged again. This went on for years.

If it wasn't for my kids and my responsibility and love for them I would probably never leave my bed, other than for my appointments. At this point the kids are used to me living on the couch and in my bed. They lived around the couch and my bed and asked me their school questions and told me about their day. But I felt isolated and detached from the rest of the world. That's OK, though. My babies are the most important.

Dr. Z recommended a biological holistic dentist, Dr. Mark McClure at the National Integrated Health Associates Center in Washington, D.C., as well as a therapist there. She wanted another set of eyes. I admire that about Dr. Z. She was always searching for new therapies and answers for her patients. She was always learning. I went. It was a huge office where everyone was hustling and bustling and always in a rush. The dentist, Dr. McClure, gave me a lot of reading material on how to arrange our home for our health. For example, the refrigerator should not be under the bedroom. He also gave me some supplements and performed some injections in my gums to take care of any infections that might have been left over from the gum grafts. He also recommended Glutathione, a very powerful antioxidant, suppositories. I saw the therapist for a while and she did some interesting treatments but insurance didn't cover her or Dr. McClure and the drive to D.C. was too much on my body, so those appointments fizzled out pretty quickly.

Then the parathyroid goes through the roof. Eventually, my labs came back with abnormally high parathyroid numbers. I so wanted this to be THE answer. The high parathyroid numbers forced me through a cascade of tests and specialists. This, again, was exhausting. Keep in mind, just lying in bed was exhausting enough. Driving to doctors and undergoing tests was enough to tip me over the edge.

Can this just be it? I so wanted this to be the answer. "Someone just take out my parathyroid and make me all better! Can you just take it out and that clear everything up?" Dr. Z sent me to an ENT in northern Virginia and he said he's seen that happen before. I didn't want to go through another surgery that didn't help, so I proceed with caution. He ordered an MRI and Sestamibi scan. The MRI shows two growths but the Sestamibi scan didn't pick them up. This indicated that the growths were too small to be what was causing the problem. Really? I was too tired to deal with this nonsense. I was frustrated with all these doctors. Why couldn't they figure it out? Why couldn't any doctor figure it out? Didn't they go to medical school? In all the books, wasn't there any answer? This was my exhaustion talking. I was actually thankful for doctors. Really. I was, and am. The doctors wanted to check my pituitary and biopsy the parathyroid. Again, I was too tired for all these decisions and appointments. I was running around to all these appointments with my head feeling like it was going to explode and feeling completely sickly. We ultimately decided on an ultrasound.

Meanwhile, my zinc went in the toilet but I was gaining some weight, which I needed. I decided to start acupuncture again. I continued chelation via IV as well as supplements Domperidone, Actigall (to prevent gall stones as my gall bladder was barely functioning), Plaquenil (to treat the autoimmune activity in my body), Coartem (another anti-parasite), thyroid cream, hormone cream, Nystatin, and IV antibiotics. I was able to get off the IV antibiotics in April and began Sucraid for congenital sucrase-isomaltase deficiency (CSID). CSID meant that I was missing the enzyme that digests sucrose. Taking Sucraid helped my digestive system tremendously...but only temporarily.

I continued to learn all I could about nutrition and diet. I learned about the power of plants and the harm that processed foods did in the body. I devoured books. I watched every video I could find. I read article after article. Matt and I had been eating better for a while, so why aren't the kids? I started talking to a few others about what I was learning. I wanted to help others even if I was not noticing drastic changes. Maybe it will help someone I came in contact with. I also didn't want my kids' world to fall apart like mine did, so I threw out all the processed foods in the pantry. They didn't know what happened to their Goldfish and cereal; I had them start trying lots of new things. We had them cut out sugar and treats. This was for their good but also out of fear I had. No matter how hard I tried I felt like I couldn't ever get enough plants into our diets. I knew how powerful and healing they were and I wanted more, more, more. Again, it was exhausting but I knew it was worth it.

In July 2012, I heard of a doctor in Richmond who specializes in TMJ and who may be able to help with my jaw and headaches. I went to see him. His office, JNT Dental, was set up just like a typical dentist's office with dental chairs. Dr. Tregaskes used a cool beam laser on my jaw and head to try to help with the pain while I waited for a mouth appliance to be made. I've had a mouth guard before. This was different. This one had a piece coming down from the top to hook the bottom jaw so that it wouldn't slide forward. It was meant to rest the jaw in its proper place. He also put me on several medications to help with the pain, as well as nerve blocks. The nerve blocks helped but only for a day. I didn't notice any improvement with the medications. Meanwhile my digestive system was getting worse and worse. Dr. Z added Yodoxin, an anti-parasite. I did better temporarily and then got worsening pelvic pain. The pain got so bad I could hardly stand it. Also, this month I followed up with the ENT and endocrinologist for the parathyroid.

The headaches continued to be SO bad. Dr. Aguilera had me do another MRI that showed nothing but migraines. He tried Midrin and Gabapentin but they didn't help. Wendy started me on some new supplements, a Glutathione nasal spray and suppositories, Rifaximin, an antibiotic, and LDN. LDN is Low Dose Naltrexone and was supposed to be HUGE for me. It is used to treat autoimmune diseases and some pain. She also added an antihistamine. I did better for a week and then miserable again. The nausea was unbearable. Dr. Aguilera increased the Gabapentin to 600 mg. daily.

My weight continued to be unstable. Through all of this that I can't control, the eating disorder had gotten stronger. Matt and I argued about it. At this point the eating disorder was so bad that I knew deep down that I needed to be in in-patient but there was no way I was going to do that. Uncle Tom stepped in to help us. As a compromise I made an appointment with a counselor, Denise, and a psychiatrist, Dr. Spanier. Denise worked in a large brick old building in downtown Fredericksburg. Dr. Spanier was at Tucker Psychiatric in Richmond, Va. Thankfully, Denise had an open room right next door to her office with toys and books that the kids could play with. We talked a lot about the eating disorder but never made real progress. We talked some about my relationship with my mother and my mother even came in for one session. I forget how it went exactly and the exact words, but I remember my jaw hitting the floor that I couldn't believe that my mother would say what she did. I remember feeling the most rejected than I ever have. I must have blocked it out. Dr. Spainer was in Richmond at a psychiatric facility. I guess I'm the judgy one here because when I walked in I remember looking around at the other patients wondering, "What are you here for? I'm glad I'm just here for an eating disorder." ;) Now that I know more about mental illnesses I am much more compassionate and open minded. Dr. Spanier put me on Lexapro, which I desperately needed. Lexapro was the turning point for my eating disorder.

This is February 2013. I still see Dr. Spanier to this day to maintain my Lexapro refills.

In January 2013, Dr. Spanier increased the Lexapro to 20 mg., which was a perfect amount for me. Wendy put me on Augmentin (a common antibiotic) and stopped Rifaximin and Depakote. I was on Depakote because it can sometimes help with migraines. At this point I was still seeing Dr. Tregaskes (the TMJ specialist) and Dr. Lim (an orthogonal chiropractor). So, I was driving like a mad woman making myself exhausted but doing it out of desperation. I wanted my life back no matter what it would take. Wendy started me on Orphenadrine, which is an antihistamine but can sometimes be helpful with migraines. I thought I noticed some improvement for a while but it may have been wishful thinking.

Chapter 6: Hang in There

In February, I met Calli Curtis through my friend Trish Mountain. When I left Calli's house in Midlothian, near Richmond, she gave me a little bag with a DVD in it and asked me if I would watch it. If you know anything about me, I get things done. So, I watched it. It was about health, and by that point, our family knew a thing or two about health. I returned it to her and didn't say much, thinking that would be the end of it. She gave me another one (eye roll). I knew through Trish that Calli was a member of the Juice Plus Company. At that point, I was too exhausted to think about what I thought was "one more thing that wasn't going to help." But she kept giving me these dang DVDs and for some reason I kept watching them and rolling my eyes, very disinterested. Eventually, one caught my attention. It showed exactly how Juice Plus was made. When I saw that it was just fruits and vegetables and it was a simple and convenient way for my family and me to get in a wide variety and quantity of plants on a daily basis I was sold. I called Calli and signed up with the company that same day that I bought the product for our family. I already knew plants were the answer. I just could never get enough! I knew my body needed more and more and more. Thank you, God, for this miracle in a capsule! And thank you, God, for giving my kids the best nutritional foundation possible!

I had already done so much research on my own about plants. However, I was thankful that the company had third party, peer reviewed, gold standard, double blind, placebo controlled studies published in leading medical journals. Why was this important when I already knew plants were good for me? Because my journey wasn't over. I would need to stand on the research. The research said these little bad boys were changing and repairing my DNA. They were protecting my cells from oxidative stress. They were turning ON MY GOOD GENES and turning OFF MY BAD GENES. This was GOOD NEWS. This made me happy.

For those of you who have not studied the relationship between nutrition and disease, you might want to take a listen to the video on YouTube by Wendy Campbell, RN.

I was still learning about health and the body and I was needing weekly hydrotherapy for my bowels. I ended up traveling to Maryland to learn more about the gut and get my certification in colon hydrotherapy. This is 100 hours of hands on, an anatomy and physiology class, CPR class, and other classroom instruction. I met some amazing people and became an I-ACT Certified Colon Hydrotherapist. I had a non-stop headache through these 10 days but I pushed through. It was important to me to continue living even in the midst of the pain. I never wanted to look back on my life and think that I missed out because of my illness.

By April, I had a few months of being very depressed and crying all the time. I was crying while driving the kids to their activities, crying while sitting in the yard watching the kids play, crying myself to sleep, etc. We eventually found out it was my thyroid. The fatigue was SO strong. I was hardly able to walk up the stairs. I remember trying to go for a walk in my neighborhood and not being able to get past my house. I was so tired. I have a new-found respect for those who deal with thyroid issues. I am SO thankful that Dr. Z has been able to get my thyroid stable even when my gut wasn't absorbing the oral thyroid medication. At this time, Dr. Z had me come in and do the Computerized Electro-Dermal Stress Analysis (CEDSA) and start supplements according to those results. The CEDSA was similar to the ZYTO scan, which tests you based on your body's energy.

I ended up having an amazing summer, especially in August. I thought, "Wow, life is SO fun when I feel good! Is this how it is for 'normal' people!? I LOVE life!" I saw a few doctors about getting my gall bladder out but we decided not to. My estrogen was a bit low but we took care of that. The headaches were less and I had more energy. I was so thankful.

I took a minute to look back and even though I was still having really hard days, weeks, months, there was some good days, weeks, months interspersed...I couldn't see it day to day but I could see it if I looked back over the years.

Unfortunately, I took a turn for the worse at the end of Sept/early Oct. 2013 and started another prescription for parasites. The fatigue and depression increased greatly. I felt very weak and sickly again like I couldn't even function. I felt the weakest I ever had and sat down and cried. I saw Dr. Z and she made a new plan.

In October 2013, I found Dr. Sneed, an osteopathic doctor in Fredericksburg and made six appointments at his office at Old Dominion Osteopathic Medicine. He tried to help me with the headaches. He used gentle maneuvers of the body. He was honest and said if they are no better after that, he couldn't help.

There were multiple times I dragged myself into the ER during a migraine episode. Normally, I would wait it out. Waiting it out meant that it would go on anywhere from a few days to three weeks. Then I would have a reprieve of a few hours to a couple of days before the next one would set in but occasionally I would see what the ER could do. I found that they could usually get the migraine to stop but it would come back in a few hours. Nevertheless, that reprieve was worth it sometimes. Especially when the migraine was so bad I couldn't think. Normally, I could push through the pain, but sometimes It was more than I could bear. The cocktails at the ER usually consisted of Benadryl, Toradol, and an anti-nausea med.

It's hard for friends and family to understand. There were years in the midst of feeling ill that I wasn't able to travel and I really don't think that my extended family understood.

I mean, I was barely making it around the house. The thought of traveling in a car for hours at a time and not having the comfort of my own home was overwhelming. Not to mention that it was hard to focus and lots of chatter and loud noises were overwhelming to me. I used to be a multi-tasking superhero but I found myself overwhelmed with simple tasks. I had to stop and think and try to refocus. When the kids asked me questions it took me long pauses to answer and I could see the frustration on their faces. But they were patient at the same time. It was becoming their normal as well.

When we did travel it was a nightmare. I battled a migraine the entire trip and walked in a daze as Matt took care of everything. I had to rest most of the time wherever our destination was. The exception was when we traveled to Hawaii. Matt had a work trip and I was determined to go with him. I felt overall better while there and my energy was up more than it had been in a long while. I was able to hike and had minimal headaches. Matt said maybe we should move to Hawaii and Wendy said that Hawaii and Colorado were the healthiest states in the U.S. We said we would do it if we could guarantee my health would stay better but we didn't know what the doctors were like in Hawaii and what if we moved there and it was a fluke.

A friend of mine was using Young Living Oils and they were helping her with some of her health problems. I was nervous about the smells because any smell triggered a migraine but I was all about natural, so I decided to at least try it. I pursued it for a good six-eight months telling myself it was working. It wasn't. They were exasperating my symptoms. I stopped and gave all the extras and diffusers to friends whom they might help.

Throughout all this I continued to take my kids to soccer, gymnastics, swimming, dance, music...I didn't want their lives to stop because mine did. I tried my hardest to keep their lives normal. I didn't want them to miss out on anything because of me. Even on the most painful days, I gritted my teeth and I made it to their games anyway. The minute I start saying, "I can't," it will start an exponential "I can't do anything" because of the pain. I didn't want that. I can. End of story.

By November 2013, my face was extremely puffy, especially my eyes. The morning was the worst. My face looked like a marshmallow. I decided to stop the homeopathics in case they were causing fluid retention. Wendy had me start Albenza again, which is a broad-spectrum antibiotic. Dr. Z had me start new homeopathics, Sinus Tone and Spectramin.

In January 2014, Dr. Z used the ZYTO again to put me on supplements, KLS, Scrofula, Gen 2, Phosphorus Oligo, Potassium Oligo and had me continue Spectramin and Sinus tone. At this point in time, I found that I couldn't think of or remember words. I felt like such crap!

A friend of mine told me about how she overcame some health challenges through Magnet therapy. What did I have to lose? It sounded kind of weird but I'd already tried some weird things, so it didn't bother me. His name was Ricardo Hidalgo and he traveled into town from Tampa, Fla. I met him along with others in a hotel room near Louden County, Va. Sounds sketchy, I know. However, I trusted this friend. She had gotten her health back on track and I was desperate. We started lining up, some other gals and me, all eager to find help. I knocked on the door and an Asian man opened the door. He was clearly in the middle of a fast food lunch. He ruffled through some papers on a desk and had me fill out some forms in the living space of the hotel. He then escorted me back to the bedroom part of the hotel room. The therapist placed magnets all over my body. He said I would feel better. I have heard that before but I figured it couldn't hurt. He also did this laser thing across any scars on my body. I left hoping it would help in some way shape or form.

In February of 2014, Dr. Z added more Progesterone, Glutathione and Theanine. I was referred to a TMJ specialist in Richmond, VCU, who put me on Zanaflex, which is a muscle relaxant. I also made an appointment with Dr. Troung, a rehabilitation specialist in Fredericksburg, VA, who began trigger point injections and recommended more massage. This month I was particularly down and depressed.

At times, I get used to it and I have adjusted to the "new normal." This is life, I think. I push through. Other times I get angry that I can't enjoy the simple things because of the pain.

In March 2014, I found a book by Dr. Buchholz at Johns Hopkins.He was actually located in Baltimore, Md., about two hours from me. The book fascinated me. It sounded just like me. I followed his migraine diet advice in the book and made an appointment. At the same time, I finished weaning from Lamictal (Dr. Spanier) and stopped all hormone cream per Dr. Spanier's advice. I got my period three times this month and my hormones were crazy. I started 23 new supplements from Dr. Z and she soon doubled the thyroid cream and added Levathyroxine. Getting my thyroid in the right place would be huge.

In May, I started Chinese herbs from Wendy (Gut Clear, Gut Bug, Antibio). These herbs ended up helping with the bloating tremendously. I also began an herb called Small Willow Flower that I read about in a book by Dr. Mitra Ray. At this point I was up for anything! A friend recommended that I See Dr. Harrison in Richmond to get another opinion on my thyroid. He wanted to put me on Armour. I feel VERY good the last week in May when on 50 Levothyroxine and 5 Cytomel but the cream is still in my system. GOOD. I start analyzing everything. This is what you do when you have a good week and you are chronically ill. However, after one week I was miserable again ~ maybe it wasn't enough thyroid med? I analyze again.

On one particularly beautiful spring day the kids were playing outside and Matt and I were enjoying the sunshine. Audrey came over to me and pointed out an all too familiar red shape on her leg. I knew it all too well from the flyers all over Dr. Z's office. I panicked. It was a bull's-eye. I called my friend Trish right away. She was also suffering from Lyme but was taking a less aggressive route than I using herbs and supplements. She lived about an hour or so south of me but we talked almost every day. I asked her what I should do and we settled on a plan of the typical three-week round of antibiotics since it was early but also to hit it with herbs. I ordered the herbs that Trish told me to and Matt took Audrey to the doctor right away. I told Matt not to leave there without three weeks and no less of Doxycycline since we were catching it early. He didn't. Audrey hated the taste of the herbs but she obliged. There were no immediate symptoms but years later she had leg aches, fatigue, and was often bloated. This was when she was a pre-teen. I took her to the doctor to see if there was some kind of explanation and, of course, the pediatrician said it was growing pains, to watch what she ate, and all her blood work was fine. I told her about the tick bite years ago and my concerns and, of course, she said that Lyme was cured with a round of antibiotics. I knew differently. I put Audrey on vitamin D to see if it would help with her energy. I knew from reading Dr. Mercola's site that vitamin D levels need to be much higher than the acceptable levels. The "growing pains" passed but she seemed to continue to deal with fatigue and digestive symptoms on and off. I mentioned to her the IVs and ozone that I had gotten and she said she didn't want to do that. For now I am respecting her wishes but I always have in the back of my mind that bull's-eye and I don't want that for my baby. It's one thing to go through a horrible illness yourself. It's a whole other story when it's your baby.

It's June 2014. I was doing colonics two days on, one day off, and thankfully it was keeping my gut happy for the most part but it's not ideal. This is not how I wanted to live. I can't travel when I'm dependent on colonics. My thyroid meds have changed a lot (switched to compounded T3/T4 16/38, a thyroid cream of 120/75 twice a day in addition to 50 Levothyroxine and 10 cytomel). Later we would switch to a suppository that would be perfect for my body and I would stay on that for years.

I drove all the way to Baltimore and saw a PA, Monica, at Johns Hopkins who started me on Linzess to see if we could get anywhere with the bowels. Unfortunately, there was no improvement from that. I felt horribly weak and sickly again by the end of the month. I was still battling the daily migraines as well as bloating that I never thought was possible.

By July, I was really down and depressed, crying all the time. I read a few books about migraines, thyroid and adrenals by Suzy Cohen. I started CoQ10 for my headaches and B2 and Rhodiola for my adrenals on my own. I was feeling very confused at this point. Why was I not getting any better? Why was my body not responding to anything? I still thought things should be progressing more quickly. I decided to see Dr. Villarreal at Embracing Health in Garrisonville to get her thoughts. Her office was beautiful, filled with plants and fountains. I wanted someone to say I was on the right track. I wanted another doctor to say, "Yes, you are doing the right things or no, you need to pivot." She agreed that I was covering my bases and didn't really have anything else to offer other than Progesterone caps. On one hand, it was encouraging but I was also still at a loss as to why I wasn't really getting anywhere. Why weren't there more answers? Why wasn't' there more progress? I didn't know at this point that Lyme took a long time to treat and I also at this time hadn't fully accepted my diagnosis. I don't know that I ever really have. Accepting that you have Lyme disease means that you are accepting that you are never really better. That you only go into remission and that you always have a chance of being sick again. I don't want to accept that.

By the end of the month it was time to see Dr. Z and do the Zyto again. Based on Dr. Z's examination, my labs and the Zyto, I started Mestenon, Cupermine, Eliquis, Bili Bile, Omega 3, and Seriphos (for adrenal support) as well as loads of enzymes and homeopathics. In between my monthly appointments with Dr. Z, I was getting weekly IVs of vitamins, minerals, homeopathics, chelation, antimicrobials, hydrogen peroxide, etc.

By August, I was beside myself. I decided I couldn't live like this anymore. By the time I saw Dr. Buchholz at Johns Hopkins in Baltimore. I was confused and desperate. As Matt drove I lay in the front seat with the seat positioned all the way back and my head throbbing. It took us about two and a half hours to get to Baltimore. I was so thankful I didn't have to drive. I wore my jean capris and a T-shirt and had all my food packed in a little cooler to adhere to his diet that I had been following. We walked up the many stone steps into the large building with columns on both sides. I followed Matt and let him lead the way.

I walked into his office and saw the little bowl of jelly beans on the counter. I slunked into one of the chairs in the waiting room and closed my eyes. When we were called back I sat in the chair near the window and laid my head back against it with my eyes closed.

Could he help me? I was scared but hopeful.

Would he have the answers? I finally got called back. I remember thinking he looked like a hippy with his long gray hair parted in the middle. I told him my story and how read his book. I told him all the things that I had tried and how nothing had worked (had nothing worked or was I just not where I wanted to be?) I told him how I was confused and frustrated I told him that his book sounded just like my headaches and could he help me? I told him how I had stuck to his diet but hadn't seen any improvement. He wanted me to stick to his diet 100% but also get off all meds and supplements except thyroid meds, CoQ10, B complex, and omegas/krill. He wondered if some of the medications and supplements I was on were exasperating my headaches. At this point I felt like I had nothing to lose. I said OK and began this August 15th. I stuck to his diet for a year while he added back in Topamax as well as Nortriptyline. There unfortunately was no improvement. The one medication I was nervous about weaning off of was the Lexapro because it has helped me so much with my eating disorder. But I had to try. I had to try something to get rid of these blasted headaches that were ruining my life. I at least had to try doing what he said or I would never know. It's important to note that going off the Lexapro was a big mistake for me. All the obsessive eating disorder thoughts came rushing back. I noticed myself turning inward and I didn't want that as a mom. I had to go back on and it was the best decision I could have made.

Hang in there.

If you have or are dealing with a chronic illness, I know it's hard. I had a family member (my own mother) tell me it was because of sin in my life. Another family member (my uncle, who is a doctor) told me it was all because of depression. One doctor told me I was just too aware of my body. Many other friends and family said insensitive things or simply seemed to not care. Give them grace. Unless someone has gone through it, they don't understand.

In September 2014, I was continuing to follow the diet by Dr. Buchholz and back to Dr. Zackrison we went. Dr. Z slightly increased the thyroid suppository. We had to switch to suppositories because my gut was not absorbing the oral thyroid medication. Thankfully, the depression lifted. So much has to do with thyroid levels! I stayed away from supplements for a time per Dr. Buccholz's advice however, she put me on Rifaximin for SIBO (small intestinal bacterial overgrowth) and Biltricide for parasites. Unfortunately, I was still dependent on colonics at this point.

I was afraid. Afraid that anything I did in normal life would hurt my body. I wanted to give my body the BEST shot. I remember I wouldn't go in pools because I knew the chlorine was absorbed through the skin and chlorine is bad for the thyroid. I soaked all my fruits and vegetables in vodka because Dr. Z said that was the best way to clean them. (By the way, I totally trust her on that one.) The point is that I was scared to eat raw fruits and vegetables because I was scared of my body being compromised by a parasite or bacteria, etc., that it wasn't strong enough to fight off.

I heard of neurofeedback and that it was helping some people with migraines. It was all over the news. I googled it and found that there were practitioners in both Richmond and Fredericksburg, both within driving distance of my house. I started neurofeedback at Dr. Catherine Ward's office in Fredericksburg. Dr. Ward is a psychotherapist who offered biofeedback, as well as other therapies. I did extensive tests before starting neurofeedback several times a week. I ended up going one hour twice a week through November 19th. I felt calmer from neurofeedback. It seemed to help the headaches while I was doing it but it wasn't lasting. I saw Dr. Mark Smith at Chiropractic Neurology in Midlothian several times as well. In addition to the neurofeedback he had me doing cranial electrotherapy stimulation (CES) daily and other brain exercises. Again, I was continuing to search for anything that might help.

In October 2014, I saw Monica, the GI PA at Johns Hopkins. It was a very long appointment and it was hard to wait so long when not feeling good. She started me on a liquid medication for my bowels and had me do a balloon test, which came back normal. Following that appointment, I went back to Dr. Buchholz this time with the kids in tow. I vaguely remembered the large buildings and how I had to drive around the winding roads to get to the back large parking lot. I held all the kids' hands and told them to look both ways as we crossed the street. We walked up the many stairs into the large lobby. We looked at the board of names to find what floor we had to go to, as the kids chatted about who would push the button to the elevator. We made our way upstairs and trudged down the hall juggling all their snacks and drinks to the waiting room. Dr. Bucholz had me start Nortriptyline 10 mg.

My body was struggling. I had a bad bout of strep that took three rounds of antibiotics to get rid of it. In my search of trying to get better I found monolaurin. A friend through Juice Plus recommended it to me. She had a friend who was suffering and had gotten better by using it.I bought a bunch and started taking several scoops a day. I finished it off and had no improvement. But I heard amazing things about it and how it was helping other people. Dr. Z put me on the Exelon patch to help move the bowels. It actually worked! This helped for several months and I was able to stop the colonics for the first time in ages! However, my body got used to it and it eventually stopped being effective. Dr. Z tried to switch me to the oral form of Exelon but I had a horrible reaction. I ended up on the floor of our hallway weak and shaking for hours on the phone with the doctor. Thankfully, we figured out it was a reaction to the medication and not something more serious. I always considered myself a smart person but all the medical stuff was overwhelming, hard to keep straight, and tough to fully understand.

I reminisce about when I felt good and could run around the yard and play soccer with the kids. I worry about never getting better. What if I am a sick grandma and can't enjoy my grandchildren? What if I never get better? I worry. But I keep trying.

I started some new injections with Dr. Z for the headaches in December. Unfortunately, they did not give me relief. At this time Dr. Spanier recommended going back on the Lexapro. I strongly agree. I noticed that when I went off the Lexapro, the eating disorder was stronger. The only way I can describe it is that my mind turned inward and started focusing on the eating disorder again. The thoughts were so much stronger. When I'm on Lexapro, the thoughts are so much less, so I can manage them.

Dr. Z is having some major success with some patients by starting them on oxygen machines. Well, oxygen never hurt anyone. We bought one. This aggravated the migraines. We can't return it. We put it in the basement. Eventually, a friend is looking for one. We pass it to her.

While at a birthday party with my girls I start chatting with another mom. I don't usually talk to strangers about my headaches but somehow it came up. She told me about a friend of hers who also had chronic headaches who is going to get surgery for them. Umm, what? She sends me the information for Dr. Ducic in McLean, Va., at the Washington Nerve Institute, and I make an appointment. He spent about three minutes with us and we found out that it's very expensive and invasive and we weren't even sure it would help. We put this on the back burner. I had another CT scan this month with oral contrast to look at the gut.

In 2015, I saw a neurologist in D.C. who took another look at my records. I honestly don't know why I saw this neurologist or how I got connected to him. He saw a disc in my neck slightly out of place. I asked him if he really thinks that is "the answer." I don't want another surgery that isn't necessary. He said probably not. He tried some numbing injections in my neck and back. It felt wonderful while it lasted. He recommended doing Botox in those areas. It wasn't covered by insurance and it was really too little time to know if that would really be lasting improvement. We decided to do Botox for the migraines with Dr. Aguilera back in

Fredericksburg. We started that in February 2015. Thankfully, the Botox helps the intensity and duration of the migraines. Finally, something is helping a little bit! I still have to avoid smells like the plague and live in my little bubble. But I am happy and thankful that the Botox seems to be breaking up the long weekly migraines a bit.

I hear of brain spotting from my cousin in New York. I google and tried to find someone in my area. I found Kathleen Hanagan in Haymarket, Va., for this treatment. I drove almost two hours to get to her office and drove in circles until I could find a parking spot. I walked into a café and then up winding stairs to the very top and down a hallway to get to her office. The walls were painted purple with lovely little decorations all over. It was an interesting treatment where she tried to find a certain spot in my brain based on the movement of my eyes. We eventually move into some counseling as well. She also told me of a doctor who does Prolozone injections in joints and also for chronic pain. I'm in. I went to see him. They were the most painful injections I have ever had but I kept getting them in hopes that they would help the migraines and neck pain. I went for six sessions and there was no improvement.

I wasn't sleeping well. I did something called EVOX (similar to the ZYTO in that it works with your energy) with Wendy and started homeopathic drops for that. I also started gaining weight. Why, I don't know. It got out of control that summer and I started freaking out. I'd never weighed this much in my life other than when I was pregnant. Others didn't understand. To them I still looked thin overall, but to me I felt huge. I gained 20 lbs. Why? I was eating the same as always. I asked the doctor. I asked multiple doctors multiple times. They didn't know. My labs looked normal. Ugh!

I was still feeling like my body had betrayed me in more ways than one. It never occurred to me that my body could let me

94

down like this. I used to be full speed at all times. Matt always gave me grace and told me it was OK if I missed a soccer game here or there or if I skipped church a Sunday or two. But it wasn't OK to me. I didn't want to miss an ounce of time with my kids! So I pushed my body as hard as I could but sometimes as hard as I could wasn't enough. It just wasn't physically possible to make my body to what it used to be able to. My kids keep me fighting. They never questioned why I was always trying to get better and was taking them to so many doctors' appointments. It was normal to them. I remembered what I used to be and I wanted that back. I never wanted to forget what the old me felt like.

I still felt awful. I was sick of having my same old symptoms. My sister-in-law recommended Dr. Anita Kloss. In Vienna, Va.She is a chiropractor who also incorporates nutritional guidance. Her desire is always to get to the root cause. She recommended an all-meat diet, of rare beef. At this point I'm like OK, whatever, sure. I tried it. What have I got to lose? I stuck with an all-meat diet for more than a year. I found multiple groups on Facebook of people having success with this and healing from chronic illnesses. What I came to believe was that it wasn't so much that it was meat that was healing them so much as that when you stick to an all-meat diet, you are eliminating sugars, processed foods, packaged foods, simple carbohydrates, etc. Just a thought. I am not a doctor. However, there are healing properties in meat like CoQ10. I did not stop my Juice Plus during this time. I would never and will never stop my Juice Plus!

In April, my T3, testosterone, progesterone, and serotonin were in the toilet again. We got my thyroid on track and I feel SO much better.

In June 2015, we went to the Mayo Clinic in Florida. It was a very long drive all the way down there. No answers. Waste of time. Huge waste of time. It was a general doctor who said I needed to be scheduled with several specialists. No kidding.

In July 2015, I tried <u>cryotherapy</u> at Help for Health in Vienna, Va. I was a bit nervous as it's not my fave thing to be cold, much less freezing. Kathy, the owner, took me to a room to change. She told me to undress to everything except my undergarments and to put on the robe provided, as well as the special socks and mittens that were also provided. After I changed I was escorted down the hall to where the chamber was. I stepped in and my whole body was submerged except for my head. I dropped the robe and gave it to Kathy. I kept moving, as it was freezing. I only had to stay in a few minutes but it feels like an eternity. The temperature is way below freezing. It was refreshing and rejuvenating. But it didn't help the pain. I went for a good 12 sessions.

Wendy started me on Questran. This is supposed to be huge. Questran is supposed to pull toxins out of your body. It is also known to cause constipation but at this point we were not worried about that since I was doing almost daily colonics anyway. I was still seeing Dr. Buchholz, Dr. Aguilera, and Dr. Spanier at this time in addition to Dr. Z.

We go back to Mayo for our specialized visits. It's a bust. They don't know anymore than we already do and have already done. On one hand, I was relieved that I was doing everything possible. On the other hand, I was discouraged that they didn't have any other answers.

By the end of 2015, I didn't know if I was a little better or just learning to function.

In January 2016, Dr. Z put me on several new supplements but I was sick and tired of IVs. I took myself off them. I didn't want that life anymore and honestly, I was functioning a bit better. At this point I wasn't thriving but I could look back over all the years and say, hey, I'm a tad better. I had been going to her office for weekly IVs for five years. I decided I wanted to believe that I was better. And going for weekly IVs didn't help that belief.

So, I stopped the IVs and only continued the monthly doctor visits. She put me on Alinia. At this point I began to switch between Dr. Z and Wendy. Dr. Z would put me on a bunch of supplements and Wendy would take me off to give my body a break. They balanced each other out well.

I got braces with Dr. Almy in Fredericksburg, Va., at Fredericksburg Orthodontics and Invisalign Center. in February 2016 to prevent any additional gum recession, jaw problems, and to even possibly help with headaches. (Dr. Buchholz and Dr. Tregaskez both recommend it). Dr. Aguilera gave me a steroid pack because the migraines were so bad this month. Dr. Z added chlorella to help detox heavy metals and a homeopathic. After a few trips to the ER for the headaches, Dr. Aguilera recommended the Jefferson Headache Center in PA. He said I was one of his most difficult patients and I need a higher level of care. Matt and I got an appointment in May 2016. Turned out they scheduled us in the wrong department, so we had to wait until September. Dr. Aguilera also gave me a calcium channel blocker and a Tryptophan injection. For a while I thought they might have been working but time would tell it was only wishful thinking. While I waited for our actual appointment at the Headache Center, I tried Dr. Berg's liver enhancement diet. I had a friend whose health really benefited from it. I didn't see any improvement but his diet really helped my husband get his weight and health back on track and he eventually completed his Health Coaching certification through Dr. Berg's program.

In September 2016, the fatigue was coming only in spurts. As long as I took an afternoon nap I seemed to be able to function fairly well. I was no longer having the severe abdominal pain and the nausea was very rare. I was no longer having the flu-like symptoms. The headaches were there but as long as I could stay away from fragrances I could manage pretty well.

I finally saw Dr. Marmura at the Jefferson Headache Center in Philadelphia in October 2016. This was a four-hour drive both there and back and we waited for hours to see him. If you have ever seen *Scandal,* the TV show, he looks like Fitz. He put me on Namenda, DHE, and Compazine. We saw him back in a few months and I was not happy. I was no better as far as the headaches went. He recommended trying their in-treatment program. We did and it was an ordeal and expensive. We did this a few times. It helped while I was there but not when I went home. While in treatment I was hooked up to an IV full of medications for several days in a row to get rid of the migraines and break them up. Dr. Marmura gave me Toradol injections, to reduce inflammation, and DHE injections to take at home. They didn't help either. He added Methergene but it gave me abdominal cramping so I stopped. It didn't help. He added Olanzapine. It doesn't help...at first. Olanzapine would be key eventually once we can get the migraines more under control.

Also in October as long as I took a nap in the afternoon my energy was musch better so I was able to join seven networking groups. I met amazing people in the community. This was so good for me for a season. I love to grow, learn, help others, and add value where I can. I grew in the areas of public speaking and had the opportunity to share Juice Plus with phenomenal businessmen and women. I am thankful for the opportunity.

I met a friend through networking who is selling the Bemer, which is a mat that you lie on throughout the day that is supposed to help with multiple ailments. It sounded cool. I like alternative things. It's rare that I find something that I haven't tried. Among many things, it's supposed to help with chronic pain and energy. My husband was skeptical. You can imagine why. I decided to try it. I have to try. What if this is the answer!? If I don't try I'll never know. Nope. Still having headaches.

It's February 2017. I followed up with Dr. Marmura. He increased my Topamax and added Midrin. We do another in-patient session in March. I'm frustrated. I let him know. I also decided to get my health coach certification. Although I already knew a lot about nutrition at this point, I wanted that certificate that proved it. I decided on Dr. Sears' program and studied my little butt off and earned my certification. By this point in time I was functioning well for me. I was struggling but not as bad as I was in 2009. I had learned to manage and manage well. I was a fighter. I also think that as a mom you do what you have to do in any circumstances.

Around this same time we moved from King George to Fredericksburg. We've lived in this house in King George for 13 years raising four kids. I can't believe all of the things we have accumulated. I realize how little it means to me and how little attachment I have to material things other than those that belong to my kids. At one point I guess I needed or wanted all of these things but now they seem insignificant. In this moment, all I want is to get healthy again. All I want is to wake up and feel the energy and pain-free life that I once knew. I used to take my pain-free days for granted. Not anymore. I think about all the healthy people out there. Do they just walk around feeling good? I can't even imagine that anymore. Do they just walk around with energy in the middle of the afternoon? Impossible, I think. I make a deal with God. If you give me my health back I will give You ALL the credit and never stop praising Your name! I know that seems silly but it was worth a try I thought.

Chapter 7: Getting Better

I look back and, overall, I am better. I am functioning. I am thankful. I can take care of my kids again and I can be a mom again. The progress has been slow but it's there. Am I not angry anymore or am I just used to it? Am I thriving? No, not yet. I'm not crazy fatigued...but I'm more tired than the average person. I can't make it through without a nap every day. I'm so thankful that the nausea and abdominal pain are gone. I still have these blasted headaches!

Early in my journey I did every test and tried every new method that might help. But now I am weary and sick of being probed and prodded. I start to decline some of the tests and procedures. There has to be a simpler way.

Matt was the most understanding and patient husband I could have asked and hoped for during the worst of the illness. Was it hard on our marriage? Yes. Did he lose the wife he married? Yes. Did it take a toll on our finances? Yes. Could he fully understand what I was going through? No. Did he question some of the treatments that I pursued? Yes. But did he always want me to find an answer and support me wholeheartedly? Yes. He would always say, "Well, you have to try it." He helped with the kids when he got home from work, drove me to doctors' appointments every chance he could get off work, and provided financially the best he could.

There were times that Matt forgot how sick I was because on the outside I looked normal. They say Lyme is an invisible disease. Matt certainly forgets now how sick I was. It's hard to remember sometimes because it was a gradual recovery and now I have so many good days. Sometimes he'll make comments about how much sleep I need and how it's abnormal. *Yes*, it is abnormal.

I have to remind him where I have been and that my body still needs extra care. Then he remembers.

During the summer 2017, I am dealing with a massive headache. I bolt up from a nap and I all of a sudden remembered Dr. Ducic! I made an appointment right away. I drove to McLean and talked to him about the migraine surgery that we had put on the back burner years ago. I am ready if he can help me. He says he has an 85% success rate. We scheduled the surgery for Sept. 26, 2017. I had the surgery and took a few weeks off of life to recover. I enjoyed that restful time with my kids. Then I had to face it - the first time I encountered a smell, the pressure, my head hurts! Yes, they are still there. Another surgery and the pain is still there. Matt is not happy. I am disappointed to say the least. I don't know if I can do this anymore. Will I ever be free from these debilitating headaches that ruin my life and steal my joy?

During fall 2017, I started to notice waves of a sickly feeling...like I have the flu or something, but I didn't. No fever, just this overall sickly feeling. I felt tired and ill. I hadn't had the flulike symptoms for years and I certainly didn't want them coming back. It would pass after a few hours or a day but then as time passed it started lasting for several days. I began to worry and got scared. I didn't want my health to go backward. I had come so far.

I was also thankful. Thankful that I was functioning and thankful for every day that I got to spend with my kids. Thankful for all the doctors who have stuck it out with me all these years and thankful for Dr. Z who had given my body all the support it needed while we fought for my life back.

In January 2018, I saw Dr. Z again, and by this time I was struggling with CRAZY fatigue. I felt like I couldn't function. Looking back, I don't think my body was able to bounce back after the surgery. I was having more of the sickly feeling and wondering what was wrong with me. I remember sitting in church and leaning over to Matt whispered desperately, "I *need* help."

Dr. Z and Wendy ordered an adrenal test and put me on some supplements in the meantime. They ordered a TON of labs. I followed up with a couple of phone consults with Wendy. Everything looked good on paper so far. Dr. Z and Wendy suggested I look for another doctor for a "fresh set of eyes." After all, they had worked with me for nine years at this point and gotten me far but there were still some humps to get over. I talked to my friend Morie. She was seeing Dr. Fletcher in Sterling. I kept this in mind until I saw Dr. Z again in March. At this point labs showed that my kidney was stressed, my hormones were out of whack, and my adrenals needed some help. She put me on a prescription and some other supplements. She liked the idea of me seeing Dr. Fletcher at Sterling Family Practice. I called Dr. Fletcher's office in Sterling, Va. They couldn't see me until July, which was months away. I felt defeated. Dr. Z gave me Dr. Fletcher's personal cell and I texted her. Dr. Fletcher's office responded that they could get me in that same week! Dr. Z said she wanted me to do visceral manipulation and ozone with Dr. Fletcher. I would follow up with Dr. Z after about three to six sessions with Dr. Fletcher.

I was hopeful but I've done this game before; the hope, will it be shattered again? I treaded lightly. I didn't want to get hopeful just to have something not work. I've done that for nine years now. I wanted to hope but I was scared too. At this same time, Dr. Aguilera and Dr Marmura told me there was a new migraine antibody shot coming out this spring. I also wanted to hope that this migraine antibody shot would be the answer but I'm also scared. I've hoped too many times already now only to have it not work.

The next day I started my new supplements from Dr. Z. I take the Moon Pearls for my hormones, the adrenal supplements, the Cytozyme KD to help my kidney that showed up stressed on my labs, the IG 26 powder for my gut. I get excited but I have two really tired days. I know it's not going to help in only two days but still....

On March 23, 2018, I saw Dr. Fletcher for the first time. She spent two hours with me doing visceral release, which means manipulating the organs. Visceral release, or visceral manipulation, is gentle movement of the organs that allows the body to release any unhealthy restrictions that is causing pain or anything that is not allowing the body to work at optimal level.

Some was painful but most was relaxing. Some was weird, like asking my body what it needs and talking to my body, but I'm not weirded out anymore. I've done weird things before out of desperation and hope. I felt somewhat better after she finished. I leave hopeful. She wants me to do 10 sessions of ozone therapy via IVs. I scheduled those with some anxiety because I am supposed to be starting my new job soon. Yes, I am going back to work full time. I never would have imagined I'd come that far. More about that in another chapter. I still didn't have a start date for the job. Dr. Fletcher said I should know by 10 sessions if the ozone therapy will help with the debilitating fatigue. Oh, God, please help. Please make it help! I spent the weekend in bed with the sickly feeling, brain fog, and crazy fatigue. I wondered how I would go back to work. I wondered how I have done it all this time and why there has been nothing that has truly helped. I wondered why my poor body hasn't been able to overcome whatever this is yet.

Ozone is O3, a more active form of oxygen. It kills all the bad stuff in the body like bacteria, viruses, fungi, and parasites. However, it is also known to strengthen the immune system and produce anti-inflammatory effects and purify the blood and lymph. When given as injections it is known to reduce pain in those particular areas, like the joints, for example (recall the

Prolozone injections that I had years ago in my neck). It is not safe to directly inhale ozone, so it must be used with precaution.

Ozone can also be applied directly to the body when infused into olive oil, drunk when infused into water, and given through IV (like I had done with Dr. Fletcher, where it is mixed with your own blood). I've also heard of it being infused through the ear and infused directly into the body rectally, as well as ozone saunas.

During March to May 2018, I underwent 12 Ozone IV sessions, two a week. It was a long trip to Sterling, Va., in traffic but I knew I had to do something. I noticed a difference after the first session. I felt a little more energy. Was it wishful thinking or was this for real? I was hopeful that my body was responding. The nurse put in an IV, extracted a full bag of blood, inserted ozone, mixed it with my blood, and put the blood back into my body. It's amazing how dark, almost black my blood is until it's mixed with the ozone and then it's a bright healthy red. I went for more sessions. I felt better and better. Thank you, God! I continued sessions with Dr. Fletcher for visceral release. My bowels started moving on their own. This was the first time in years that I didn't have to use the colonic/hydrotherapy device. I thank God because little do I know that in the near future I will have to travel every weekend to Durham, N.C., to visit my daughter in the Veritas treatment center. Depending on colonics made it very hard to travel.

It's summer 2018. This is the most normal I have felt in 10 years! I was about to start working full time in August. I enjoyed my summer with the kids, an almost normal mom, still suffering from migraines but that was my normal. Never in a million years would I have expected that I would even have been able to consider going back to work full time. I was even able to make a few trips to Kings Dominion in Doswell, Va., with the kids. I always get anxious about big day trips like that because I don't know if I

105

will feel good or bad. But I made it through and had a great time. I am SO thankful. I am feeling stronger and healthier. My energy is up and the flulike symptoms have gone.

It's August 2018. Aimovig comes on the market, the new antibody migraine treatment that I have been waiting for. We had to jump through hoops with insurance to get me started on it. Thankfully, this brings the headaches down to only twice a week. Can you believe it!? I went from daily migraines for years to only twice a week!? I'm thrilled! Unfortunately, after a few months of being on it, insurance decided to say they won't cover that because I'm on Botox for the migraines. Then they said they didn't think the Botox was helping me "enough," so they weren't going to cover that anymore. I felt like I was being punched in the stomach. Really? I finally have something that is reducing my headaches and you are going to take it away? My neurologist and I appealed twice over a period of several months and eventually get me back on both the Aimovig and Botox.

Along the way I learned about positive and negative self-talk and the way we think about ourselves. During the worst of the eating disorder, I did my fair share of self-hatred.

I learned that the way we talk to ourselves releases positive or negative energy and effects on our bodies. Let's face it, it's hard to control all our thoughts during the day, but it's not so hard to make habits like a gratitude journal or to go to bed at night saying things like, "I'm so happy and grateful for…this that and the other." Going to bed on a positive note is good for the body physically, mentally, and emotionally.

From January to May 2019, I notice how tired I am. I was working full time and had to go to bed very early. I am very aware of where I have been. I know I have to take care of myself. I can't feel guilty for that. I have the fear in the back of my mind that if I don't take care of myself I could go back there. It's been 10 years since it all started and I can't even believe how bad it used to be. I just went for a few ozone tune ups. I bought an ozone device to have at home because I know it helped me so much. I can't believe I can function now and work full time. I'm not saying it's easy. I am still more tired than the average person and have to be very careful with my schedule, that it's not too draining. But I can look back and see how far I have come. I can get up every morning and work a full-time job and go most weeks with only mild headaches and some mildly unusual fatigue. I think back to my worst years and wonder if I had known I would have come this far would it have been easier to get through. But life is full of unknowns and we have to do the best we can.

I just saw my neurologist in Pennsylvania and he said there are new migraine medications coming out this summer that have been in the works since the '90s. I thank God for the timing. I see him in the fall to start trying some of them to hopefully get these headaches down to even less than two a week. The big difference now is that not only are the migraines less often and less intense but when I do get a migraine I can take both Olanzapine and Naproxen and usually get rid of it within a day. My number one trigger is still fragrances. It is very hard for me to be in public places. We are still completely fragrance free in our home.

On November 14th, 2019, Matt and I drove up to PA again for my bi-annual check in with Dr. Marmura at the Jefferson Headache Center. I had had a really good stretch of about 9 months since the combination of the Aimovig and the Botox but the last few months I felt like I've been in a rut. I shared this with him and he said it can be normal to fall into a rut after a good stretch so that was good to hear. I didn't want to go backwards for good. He said there were a few new medications on the market similar to Aimovig but we both agreed it wasn't worth rocking the boat by trying them when it seemed Aimovig had helped so much. The most important thing was getting me out of this rut. We agreed on a plan that involved being on a short- term dose of Prednisone, a short term dose of a medication called

Methergene and trying a new device that just came on the market called QuickCare. I had been on Methergene before but it had given me abdominal cramps so we stopped it. However, he wanted me to give it another try. The QuickCare devise goes on the arm and is controlled by an app on the phone. Dr. Marmura said that the people who have tried it either love it or say it doesn't work at all. It's either all or nothing. I'm hoping for all. We scheduled my usual appointment in 6 months for which he said several more oral rescue drugs will hopefully be on the market.

Overall, I am a functioning adult again. I am thankful to all the doctors who have cared for me through this and for my friends who have listened and not judged, for my husband who has supported me emotionally and financially through this, and I want to encourage anyone who is going through a trial to press on and not give up because, for most, there IS a light at the end. You will NOT always be in the trial. It is hard while you are in it and it seems like it will never end. I was angry and I questioned God and I yelled at God but things change and it doesn't stay the same forever. The one thing I did was never gave up. I kept seeking answers and I hope you do, too. I have not stopped seeking treatments. I am still looking for the next level of health. I still remember the days when I felt on top of the world. I don't know if I will ever get back to that point but I keep seeking.

Today, I can function with only a few supplements and some ozone boosting. I take my Juice Plus, triple the recommended amount, and a vitamin D supplement for my bones. My bones were suffering from osteopenia and now my spine is back in the normal range and my hips are still a little weak but are building back bone. I take my thyroid medication and Lexapro daily. I make sure I get PLENTY of sleep and am very protective of my sleep time. I have to make sure I never plan too much in one day. I have to avoid stores and places with too many people or I know I will get a migraine. However, if I manage my environment right, I can go a week with only a mild headache. I can pretty much live a normal life. When I do get a migraine, I can take my Naproxen and Olanzapine and pretty much knock it out. That makes me SO excited. I could never do that before. They used to set in and set in for weeks. I rely heavily on my Botox injections every three months and my Aimovig injection every month to keep the migraines at bay. I also take Topamax still daily for the migraines. I give myself regular Ozone tune ups via IV with Dr. Fletcher, as well as use my own ozone generator at home. I know by body needs it. I take Mag07 to keep my bowels going. Mag07 is not regular magnesium. It helps to ozonate the bowels. You can find it on Amazon or at the Vitamin Shoppe. I am still on my Lexapro for the eating disorder and I will take that for life. The big difference is that I wake up expecting to feel good and live a normal life.

I was driving in the car today and realized I had been focusing on the negative lately. I had been whining about my job and focusing on ways that I wasn't happy. I all of the sudden bolted up in my seat, wide eyed. How DARE I complain! How dare I focus on the negative! Look at where I have been! Look at how far I have come! Had I forgotten? Getting better has been so gradual that I was taking all these good days for granted. I took a moment to remember how bad it was and how I used to thank God for just one good day without a headache. I let my mind go back to the days when I just lay around in pain wishing and hoping to just be able to function again and here I was, doing just that, but instead of being happy for getting my life back, I had forgotten. I had forgotten not only how bad it was but I had forgotten to be thankful and joyful and happy and to enjoy life! I thought back to that time in August when I felt good in the midst of the storm and I realized how fun life was just because I felt good. THAT is what I wanted. That is what I wanted to remember and never forget. I thanked God for the wake-up call. Oh, God! Let me never take these good precious days you have given me for granted! Is that what you wanted to teach me through all this,

God? Jeez. That was a lot to go through to teach me that. I wonder often what God wanted to teach me through all that hardship and all that pain. I'm thankful that I learned about good nutrition so that I can give my kids a better nutritional foundation. I am thankful that I learned to be more sympathetic to those struggling with any kind of chronic pain...or any pain for that matter. I'm thankful that I learned to let go of things in life and to not try to have so much control. There are a lot of little things that I learned. Does that mean I'm thankful to have gone through those 10 years of pain and trial? Not so sure but it's God's way, not mine.

I saw a quote on Instagram the other day: A healthy person has many dreams, a sick person has one. When I was sick, nothing mattered. Nothing mattered but getting better. I lost interest in everything that mattered to me other than my family and getting better. Outings, my appearance, and keeping the house spotless, all of those things just seemed silly and pointless. Why did I ever care about that, I asked myself? I just wanted to get better for me and my family. Now, I get frustrated with things like traffic. Little tiny things like traffic that don't matter and I have to remind myself, "Ariel, you used to be in bed in pain all the time. You GET to sit in traffic! You GET to go to work." Getting better has been so gradual that it's easy to take it for granted but when I stop and remember from where I came, I am SO thankful!

There are a few doctors who have been most prominent and have really stuck with me through this whole process.

I want to thank Doctor Z, who really dug deep to the root cause and nourished my body at the same time as cleansing it. She took the time to really know my body and handle it as an individual case and know it as a whole. She thought outside the box and I loved that she was an M.D. but also very alternative, so that she could treat me from both angles.

I'm thankful that she was able to get my body in a place where I could function again and she pointed me in the direction of Dr. Fletcher, even though Dr. Fletcher only played a small role in how *frequently* I saw her, she played a huge role in that she got me over the hump of the chronic fatigue at the end and the huge hump of getting my bowels moving again. It's hard to know if that would have been possible if I hadn't been preparing my body for that all those years with Dr. Z.

I am thankful for my neurologist Dr. Aguilera, who never gave up on me and persistently worked to find treatments to get the headaches under control and who continues to work with me alongside Dr. Marmura at the Jefferson Headache Center. I honestly do not know how I used to cope or make it through day to day with a migraine every day. I spoke with Dr. Aguilera about this the other day and he said, "because you had to." That's right, because I had to. I had four little ones depending on me every day. Now when I get one I take my medication and sleep it off. But when I was getting them every day and had four littles to care for, sleeping every day wasn't an option. I have no idea how I did it other than my personality to get through and being a mom you just do what you have to do in the present moment. Dr. Aguilera not only stuck with me but he fought with insurance to keep me on Botox and Aimovig. I am thankful for both him and Dr. Maurmura for looking ahead to new medications that are coming out and giving me hope that one day I can live even more free from these blasted headaches.

Mostly, I thank God for putting these doctors in my path. He knew whom and what I needed. He knew my body better than anyone and He is the ultimate healer. Would I have wanted to be healed faster? Ummm, yes. Would I like to have no headaches now? Ummm, yes. But we live in a fallen world and it all comes back to trust. His ways are perfect. His plan is good and there are so many ways I can see His care for me.

If you are struggling with a chronic illness, don't give up. I remember asking God, "Will you just tell me if I am going to get better or not? Because if I'm not going to get better then I can just stop trying so hard!" But imagine if I had stopped trying, as exhausting as that was in and of itself. I'd have missed out on getting my life back. Keep on keeping on.

Chapter 8: What the Kids Remember

Karis was 8 months old when it started. She is 11 now (2019).

"I remember that we would go to Adee's house a lot and that Mom would always be in bed and we would constantly be going places every day for doctors appointments' and stuff and it would take like one and two hours to get there. We wouldn't really go anywhere else besides that. I didn't really know what was happening because I was so little. It was kind of normal because I just did what little kids did like tag along. I remember we used to make funny names for all the doctors and laugh when we heard their real names. I used to think making Mommy's capsules was fun. I was fine with Mom's IVs because of the snack machine and Mom would always give us money for the snacks. But I did think when Mom had that thing at home where she had to carry it everywhere, that was weird. (She is referring to when I had a PICC line at home and had the IV in.) And also, that lady that used to pick you up was weird. Basically, you are better but you still have some headaches. "

Connor was 1½ when I got sick and is 12 now.

"I remember Mom taking a lot of naps and we got dragged along to a ton of doctors' appointments and every day we went to a new one. Some days we would skip school because of doctors' appointments. We still did soccer and I remember Mom couldn't go anywhere because of smells, so Dad had to do all the shopping and stuff. It seemed kind of normal because it was all I was used to but I remember Mom would just rest a lot. I felt like I didn't miss anything because that was what I was used to."

Audrey was 3 when it started and is 14 now.

"I think Mom is definitely a lot better now than she used to be even though she still gets headaches and has to take lots of medicine that makes her tired. When we were younger Mom had what felt like a million doctors' appointments. I remember driving to Washington, D.C. and Richmond every week at one point. Also, when we kids were little we used to make names for the different doctors' offices. Some names were, "The Far Away Doctor," "The IV Doctor," and "The Place with Snacks," etc. A lot of times while Mom was away we'd spend the day at our grandparents' house and do our school there (since we are homeschooled). Other times we would pack our school work to do on the road. I don't remember if we complained a lot or not (I'm sure we did) but nevertheless we had fun and joked, too.

"For a while I would get frustrated 'cause I didn't understand why I couldn't have good hair products that had a fragrance or why we couldn't paint our nails at our house with our friends or why we couldn't use nice smelling laundry detergents because it would give Mom a headache. It seemed like such a small thing but it would give Mom a headache that would last for days. Mom would sleep a lot, too, for hours every day. It was normal, though: Go to doctors or grandma's house and bring our school work, go home, Mom takes a nap, then whatever else we did in the evening. I definitely know that Mom still has days she doesn't feel good and it's also not as bad as it used to be. I won't even understand fully but sometimes when I get a headache or stomachache I think, "Wow, Mom used to feel like this every day." She's an amazing mom and despite what she's been through she still puts us first. Love you, Mom!"

Tyler was 5 when it began and is 16 now.

"It was so long ago. I remember that Mom used to pretty much be asleep all day. We would just go to doctors' appointments all the time. I would worry about Mom. I wanted her to get better. I didn't know when that was going to happen. I mean, we pretty much kept up with life. We were so little. School was hard since sometimes Mom couldn't always answer questions. Mom stopped going to most of her doctors' appointments once she started doing JP. She didn't have headaches every single day and didn't take naps every single day probably when I was around 13. She wasn't 100% better but it was good to see that she wasn't as sick. Now she doesn't really have headaches as often unless she smells something. She doesn't really say that she feels sick very often anymore."

For those of you in a chronic illness who are trying to raise children, I know it's hard. I want to encourage you – my children are fine. I worried and had mom guilt and was scared that it would affect them, but guess what? They are fine and are perfectly normal functioning children. I wouldn't change anything about them. Do the best you can, pray and seek direction from the Lord for their school and for their lives. He is taking care of them just like He is taking care of you. He is molding them and shaping them and making them more like Christ through this just like He is working on your heart.

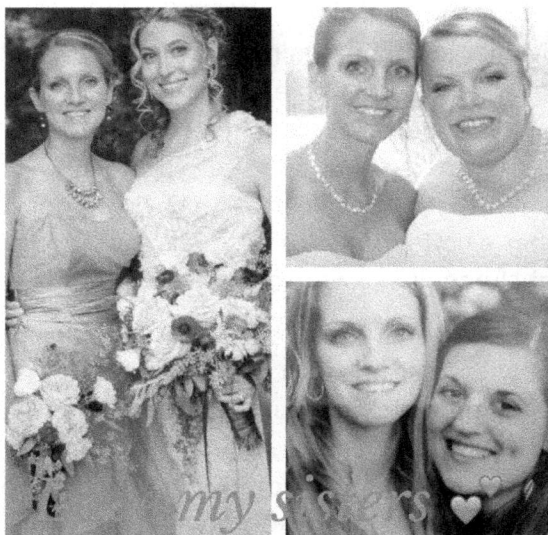

Collage of me with my three sisters

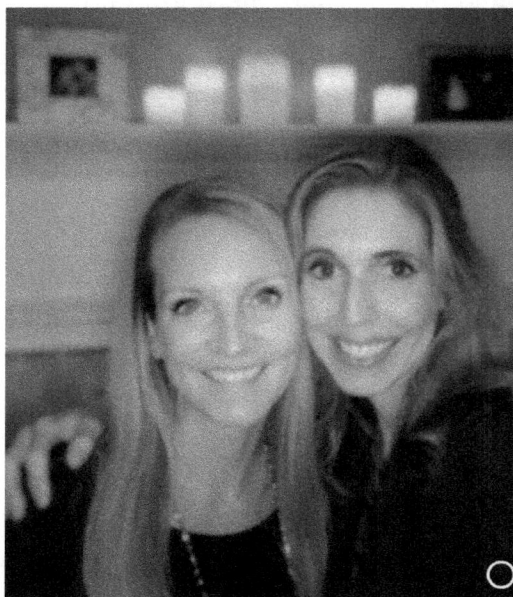

Visiting my BFF in VA Beach

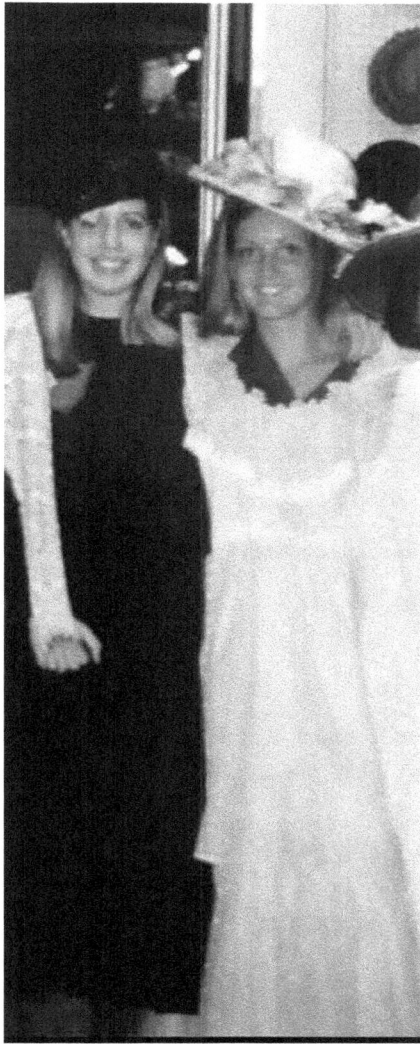

1997 with my BFF Stephanie; dressing up at a consignment shop in downtown Fredericksburg

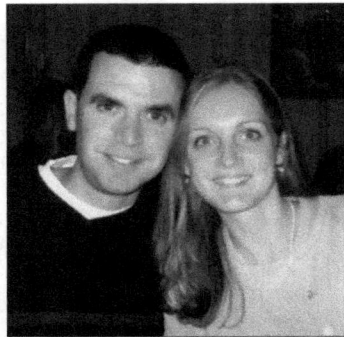
2007 at a friend's wedding

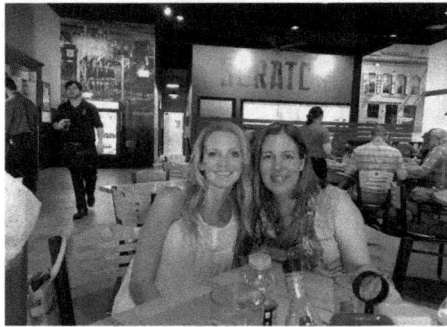
Celebrating my 39th birthday with good friend Kristin

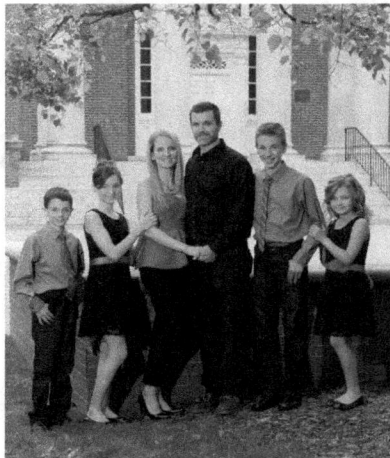
Family Picture 2017 at UMW

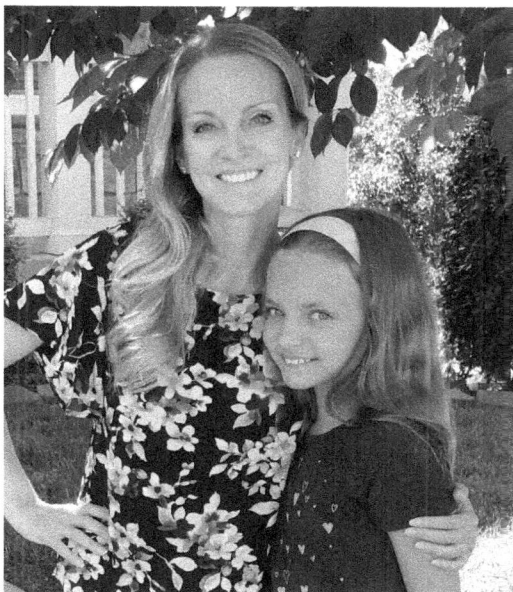

With my daughter Karis on my 40th Birthday

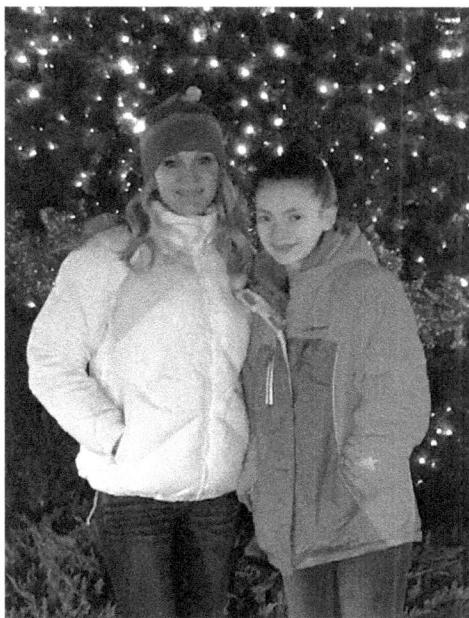

With my daughter Audrey at Christmas time 2017

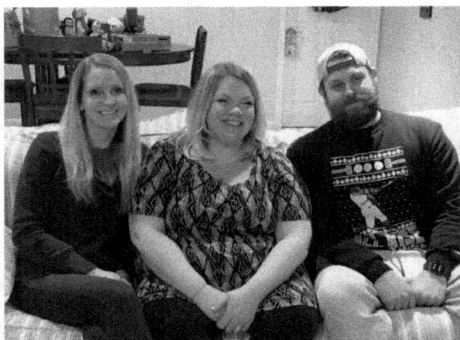
My sister Julianne and brother Zack; Christmas 2018

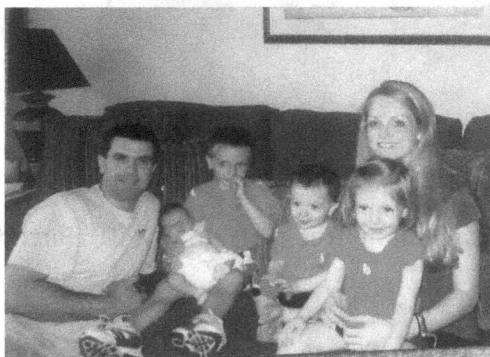
Family picture in 2008 at Matt's parent's house

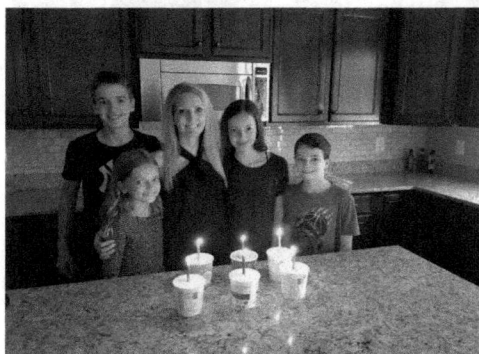
Celebrating my 38th Birthday

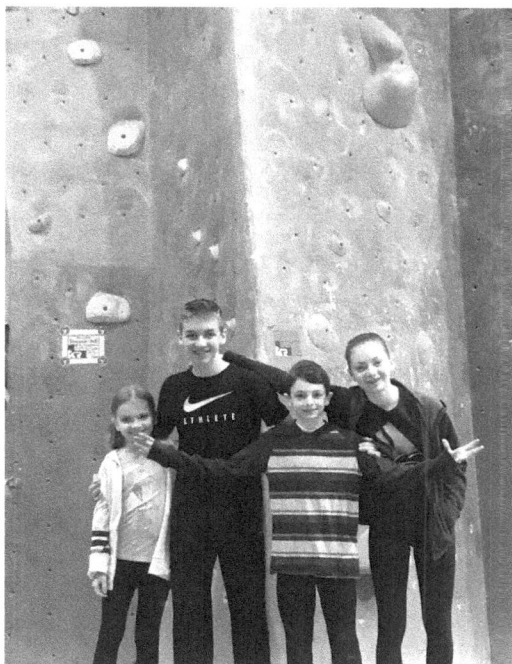

Tyler, Audrey, Connor and Karis rock climbing in Northern VA

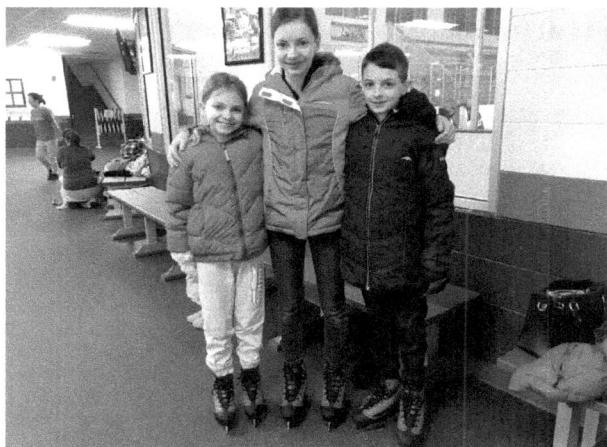

Ice Skating in Northern VA with Karis, Connor and Audrey

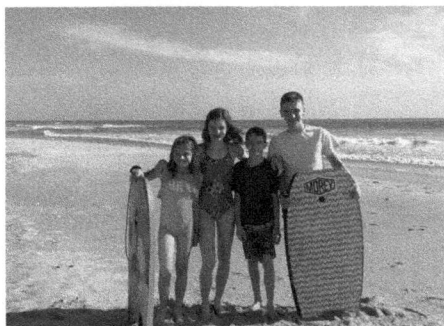

Vacationing in Outer Banks NC; An every year tradition

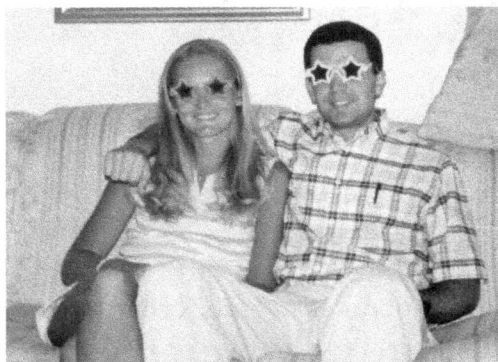

Matt and I at my Mother and Stepfather's house the summer after we got engaged

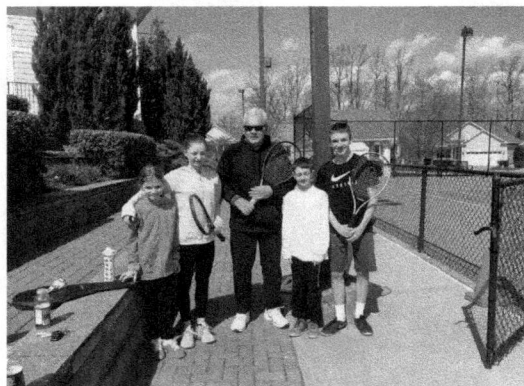

Playing tennis with my Dad

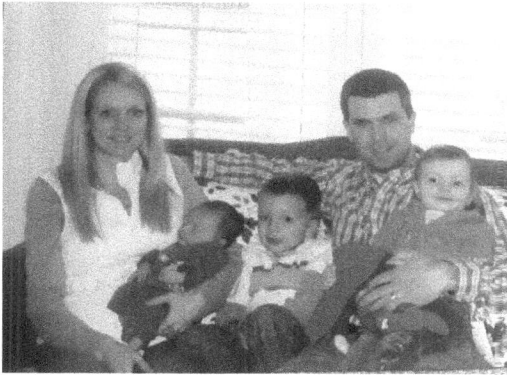
Family picture in 2007 at Matt's parent's house

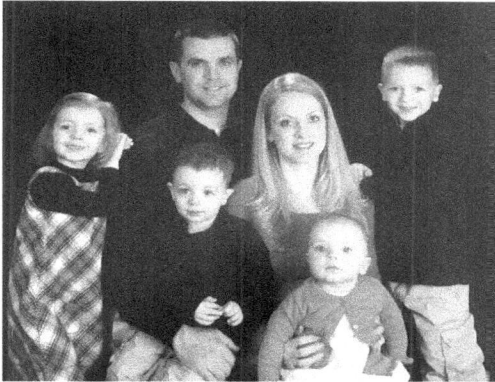
Family picture after Karis was born; 2008

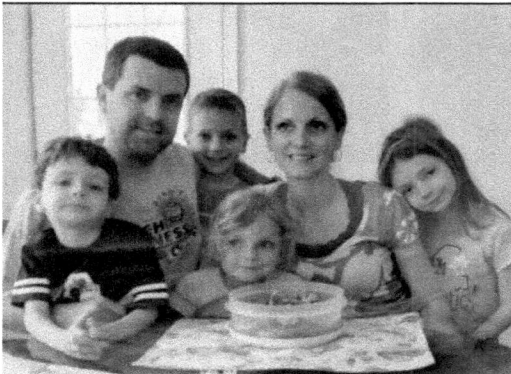
Family picture at my most sickly time

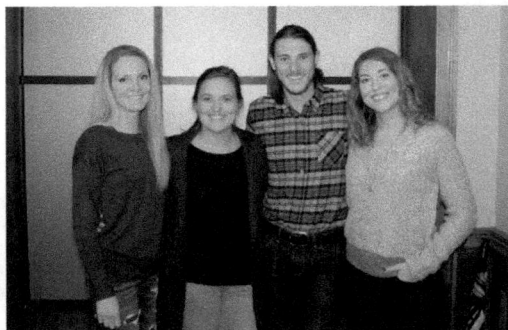

My siblings Jenna, Lindsey and Aaron

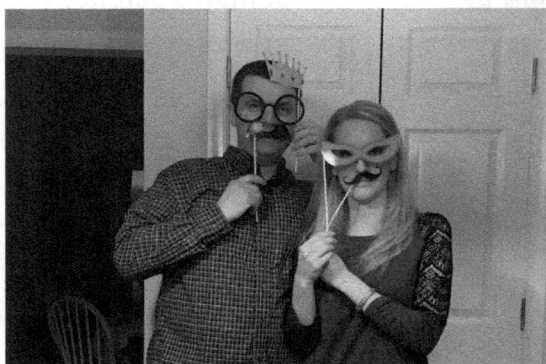

Matt and I New Years Eve 2018 spent with our friends the Garcia's

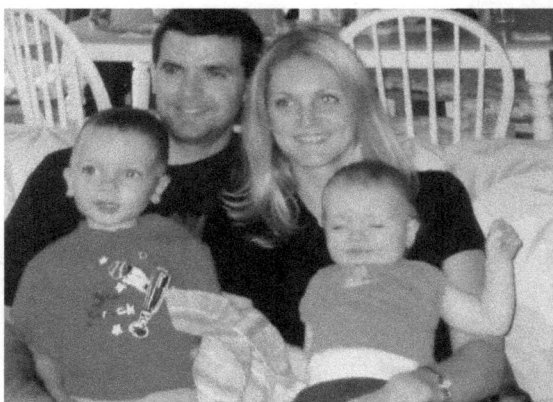

Matt, Ariel, Tyler and Audrey 2006

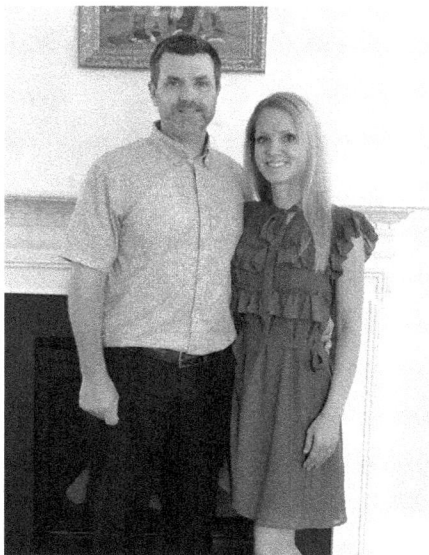

Matt and Ariel 2018; Ariel's 39th Birthday

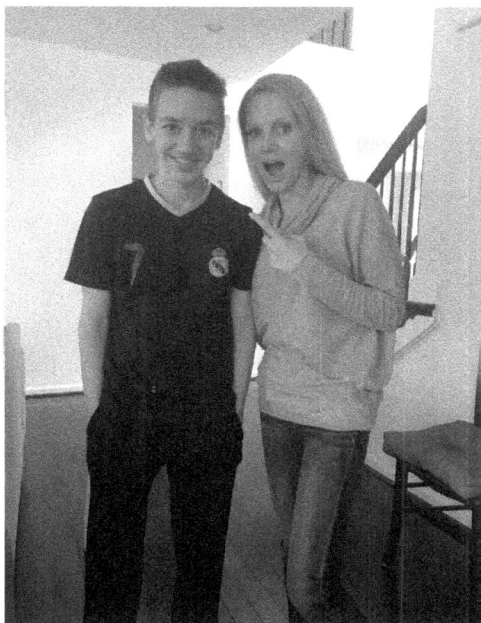

Excited for Tyler to get his braces off; 14 years old

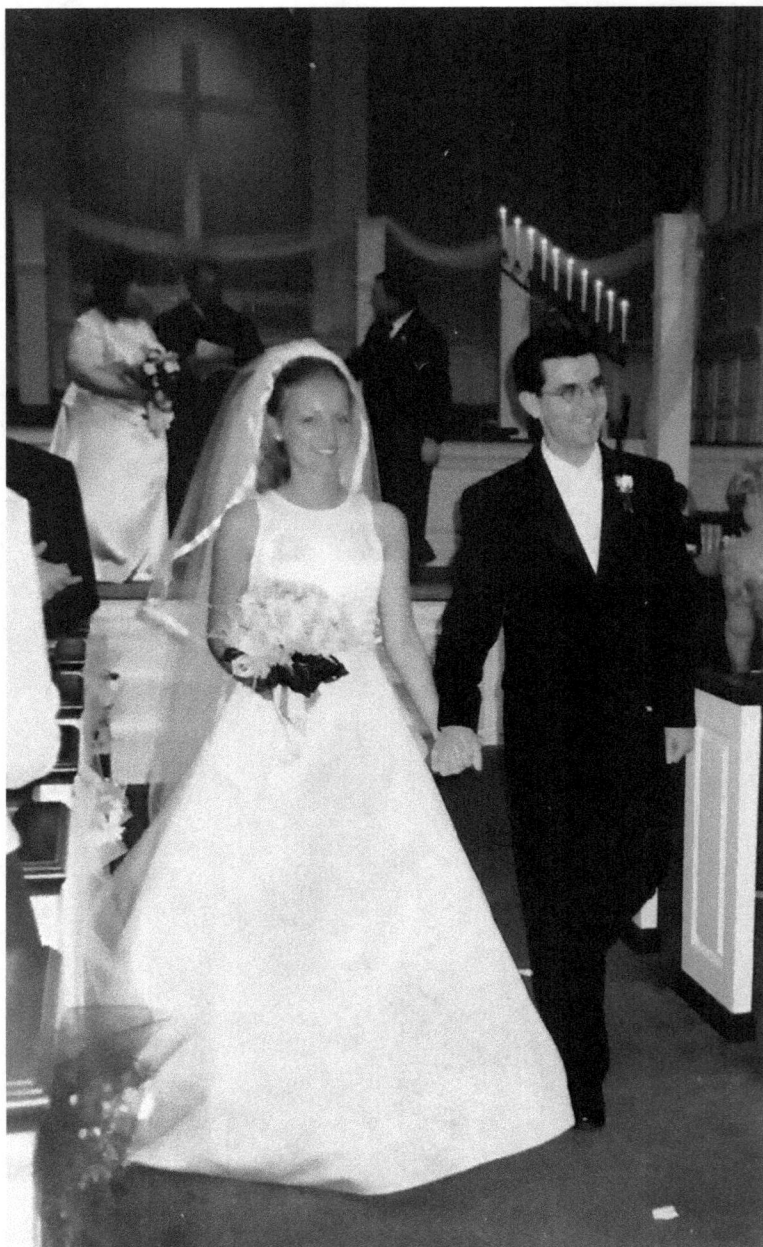

Our Wedding

Chapter 9: Going Back to Work

Never in a million years did I think I'd go back to work. I'd been home with the kids for 15 years and loved every minute of it. But we had accumulated some debt and I felt like it was holding us back. What really did it for me was finding a vacation deal online and Matt saying, no, not until we finished paying off our debt. What? Matt never said no to me. That was it. I wanted to pay off our debt as fast as possible. We were paying it off slowly but that wasn't good enough. I started thinking about going back to work for a year, paying it off, and then coming back home to the kids. I thought about maybe going back to teaching...or maybe looking for an administrative position since I didn't want the paperwork that went with teaching. I started looking for things that I could do from home.

At that time, I was still struggling with headaches and crazy fatigue. I had no idea how I would work full time. But I always had a lot of determination in me. I always believed I could do anything I put my mind to. Just like I believed I could get better, otherwise why would I have tried so many treatments!? Even so, I still wasn't totally sold on going back to work...I was really emotional about it and wasn't sure how to work it all out.

My husband ran into someone at work in Dahlgren, VA who liked to hire math majors because of their attention to detail. He asked for my résumé. Really? We had just moved to Fredericksburg and I really didn't want to drive all the way back to Dahlgren, Va., for work. Nonetheless, I gave him my résumé. I got an email the next day asking if I could meet for an interview. I guessed it couldn't hurt. He offered me the job that same day. I was nervous but how could I turn down such an amazing opportunity. I mean, I thought moms who have been home for 15 years don't get opportunities like this. I told him it would be a big learning curve. He said that would be OK. I ended up taking the job in March 2018, although my start date wasn't until August of that year. I'd be working in Dahlgren, Va., at the Navel Surface Warfare Center.

In the months leading up to my start date the fatigue had gotten worse and worse following the headache surgery, so I was nervous but I knew I could do it. Thank God Dr. Z sent me to Dr. Fletcher because Dr. Fletcher's ozone therapy was exactly what I need to get my energy on track. This was the first time in nine years that I felt almost like a normal person again. Praise God!

I started working Aug. 6, 2018. The first month was unbearable. All the new smells were triggering my migraines. I pushed through and learned whom to avoid (who smelled) and when to avoid the bathrooms (when they were being cleaned and smelled like cleaning products). When I first started working I liked the newness of it. I liked having something to get up to every morning. I liked feeling that I had a new purpose. I also love to learn and grow, so I looked forward to that. As time went on I missed my kids. I began to have some resentment. I think I directed it to Matt because he made comments about him wanting me to work long term when the original plan was to only work a year. After all we had four kids to put through college and then weddings, all four to add to car insurance, two more to put through braces, the list goes on. If you have kids I don't have to tell you! When would the expenses end? We had many unexpected expenses that first year of me working and so we were paying off debt slower than expected. This frustrated me beyond belief because this wasn't the plan. Remember, I like to be in control! I tried to counteract that with being grateful for my job and even more importantly with being grateful that I was well enough to work full time. I never would have imagined in a million years that I would get to this place but I had always been hopeful.

I thanked God every day for how He took care of me at work. He put me in an office suite with three people who didn't wear fragrances! The person who trained me didn't smell at all, not even of detergent like so many people do! God was protecting me! Even when they hired someone new for me to train, she was very understanding of my sensitivity to fragrances and did her best not to wear anything that would bother me! Thank you, God, for watching over your little girl.

Dr. Marmura, my neurologist at the Jefferson Headache Center, cautioned me now that I was doing so much better, to focus on things that I enjoyed and maybe not just going back to work. I knew he was right but I felt stuck at work. This was not to say that work was a bad thing. I love to learn new things and I just can't help myself in wanting to move up. I'd love to move into line management and I was getting good feedback. I've been given amazing opportunities at work already and for that I am so grateful. But I wanted to make sure that I was spending quality time with my kids. I didn't want to have any regrets. I'd had enough of those. I have mom guilt all the time and I know that is something working moms deal with frequently. I started to think about what I wanted in life and what I would be doing if I wasn't working. Was Dr. Marmura right? But I didn't feel like I had that option. I needed to help provide for my kids financially. I wanted them to have choices in life and choices cost money.

I'm thankful for what my job provides. I want to say "YES" to my kids. It's not about the money in and of itself but it's about what you can do with it. Money gives you choices and I want to give my kids freedom and choices along every path of their lives mostly because I didn't have choices.

When I was little I was obsessive over cleaning my tennis shoes. My family teased me and thought it was just because I liked clean shoes. Really it was because I wanted to take care of those shoes because I didn't know when or where the next ones were coming from. I remember not having enough outfits to get through one full week. I started buying my own toiletries in high school and buying some of my own clothes with my own money I got from babysitting in middle school and high school. I'm not saying poor me. And I'm certainly not saying we didn't have food on the table. We lived a certain way because that is what my parents chose. When I became an adult, I caught myself buying multiple of the same shirt or pants or shoes. Weird, I know. When I got to the bottom of it I realized it was because it was rooted in my childhood. I was worried that when one wore out where would the next one come from? I had to remind myself as an adult we had money. I was going to be OK. It's crazy how things stick with you.

Don't get me wrong. I am SO thankful that I got to stay home with my kids for 15 years. But I don't want to home school anymore. I'm not one of those moms who is passionate about home schooling. I just like to have fun with my kids. I just like to spend time with them. So, when they were little, being home with them was the way I could be their best mom. Now that they are older, this is the way I can be their best mom.

And I'm not judging any mom out there. Being a mom is hard and every mom has to choose and do what is best for them and their family! A huge shout out to all the moms out there! What I have found as a working mom is that what I really want is to be a working mom at home. I love to be busy and productive but I also love being around my kids. They don't need me in the same way that they did when they were little. If I stayed home now without working I would be bored out of my mind, but I love to be around them and busy with tasks at the same time, so that on little breaks I can spend time with them and when they do need me I am there. Working from home, doing something similar to what I do now but at home, is my dream now. I am thankful that I have a job that allows me to do that one day a week and maybe one day I will have a job that allows me to do that even more often.

Because I'm still more tired than the average person I have to go to bed VERY early in order to be able to handle working. But I have to take care of myself. I don't ever want to go back to what it was. I am the most normal now than I have been in 10 years. I never want to be sick again if I can help it.

I'm very aware of where my health has been. I bought an air purifier for our office as well as a rock salt lamp, both to purify the air. I also bought some plants that are known to clean the air. It may sound silly but I am still thinking of ways to help my health in any way that I can.

Work in and of itself has been challenging. It was initially a hard transition. There were many days that there wasn't enough work for me to do and I like to be busy, so the days were long. I took over for someone who retired and it was hard for him to let go of the work. This meant I wasn't trained or prepared like I should have been. I wasn't even sure I liked the work. It wasn't exactly what I went to school for or was passionate about. I had to learn the significance of what I was doing. There were days I was overwhelmed, days I was frustrated, days I wanted to quit and also days that I enjoyed what I was doing. I love the people that I work with. It's such a mixture. I am not a quitter. On the hard days, my husband wanted to fix it and have me look for something else. But I don't give up on things. I like to put in my all. I like to really understand things and give it time before I decide I've had enough. I've learned that about myself. I look ahead. I see opportunity. I never want to look back and have regrets if I can help it. Like I've said before, I've had enough of that. I persevere. I am a hard worker and I don't jump ship. I think of the quote that says, "I want to inspire people. I want someone to look at me and say, 'because of you I didn't give up.'"

If sharing my story somehow helps someone to not give up then it will all be worth it.

I've been at work for a year now and I'm glad I didn't give up. The person that I took over for has retired, and that has removed a lot of stress. Things are starting to click for me and I love the sense of purpose. I can see room for growth and opportunity and I love to take on more responsibility. Again, I trust that God gave me this job and am thankful. I am thankful and look forward to working here many more years!

When I was sick, I asked God if He would give me many more bountiful years after my sickness was all over and I believe He is. Not only am I extremely grateful for the opportunities that I have had at my current job but I am amazed every day that I can get out of bed, feel good and work a fulltime job. I am thankful for the many doors that God is opening that are related to my fulltime job and other part time opportunities that He is blessing me with.

Chapter 10: The Eating Disorder

Professionals say that an eating disorder is a combination of genetics, a biological factor, and an environmental trigger. At 18 years old, in fall 1997, I broke up with a boyfriend of 1½ years because I 100% believed that God was telling me to. There was nothing wrong with our relationship. In fact, it was wonderful. It broke my heart to follow through with it and at that time it was the most painful thing I had ever had to go through. I didn't realize it until after the fact but being in that relationship was the first time I felt completely whole and completely secure…and then I lost it. And I lost myself.

But I had no idea that it would trigger an eating disorder. I don't even think I knew at that time what an eating disorder really was. I guess that breakup was the trigger that started the eating disorder that would go on for 22-plus years.

Before the eating disorder started, I had always been very thin and able to eat anything I wanted without gaining an ounce. I'd never thought twice about what I'd ate or how much. A focus on food was completely brand new to me. It started with eating more than usual and not being able to take my mind off of food. The thoughts were constant and I would list the restaurants out in my mind that I would try to eat at that week. I'd pile my plates up during the day, way more than I'd normally eat. Looking back, I was trying to fill an emotional hole. Then the binge eating started. I'd eat until I felt sick and then I'd keep eating some more. I'd often do this in secret and then struggle with guilt and shame afterward. It would be anywhere from an entire carton of ice cream and whole pan of brownies to odd concoctions like nuts with icing spread on them. It was often sweets that I craved but it could be anything. I would try to "do better" the next day but I couldn't stop thinking about food and whenever I was alone the urge got 100x stronger, I couldn't stop myself and then I was flooded with the feelings of guilt and shame all over again. I would go through everyday feeling so full that my stomach was stretched out farther than I thought it was even able to go but even still I wanted more food. I was out of control but I couldn't stop it. I had no idea what was happening. All I knew was that I couldn't stop thinking about food or when the next meal would be and I would binge eat in secret until I felt sick. This went on for a good year. When I expressed what was going on to my parents (Mom and my stepdad) they would blow it off. I remember my stepdad saying, "Well, everyone overeats sometimes." This wasn't "overeating sometimes."

I tried to read my Bible and pray but it felt like God wasn't helping me. Again, I tried to tell my mother and step father but they had no advice to offer. They weren't getting it. I remember them telling me to "confess" it to them every time I binged as if that was sin. So, I did, every time I binged but that wasn't helping the problem. Sometimes I would binge at the house I grew up in and then in desperation to stop or to get away from it I would drive to my dad's house but then there would be food there or they'd be sitting down to eat dinner and so I'd eat again. Not because I wanted to, but because I couldn't' stop thinking of food. I was so desperate for help.

I was longing for the bingeing to stop. I remember our church was having a day of fasting and prayer, so I decided to fast the entire day. This was my first time going without food. The only way I knew to get a hold of the bingeing was to stop eating. I had to do something. So I really put my mind to it. I started to swing back in the other direction and began to starve myself. Let's say, I was trying to starve myself. The bingeing didn't fully go away. I ate less and less and less until my body was starving and then I would binge. Then I would feel so guilty from the binge that I would starve myself again until the next binge came along. I remember going a week with only eating two little rolls. I didn't know how else to get control of the binge eating. I remember chewing gum to try to avoid eating and starving as long as I could take it. The problem is that I would starve and starve and starve until I was so hungry I would binge. Then I would feel guilty and starve myself again. The cycle would continue.

I remember not eating for a day or two and then going to buy a full-on cake at the grocery store. I ate the whole thing secretly in my car. Situations like this were common. I would then be so disgusted with myself that I would vow not to eat anything the next day to make up for it. That, or I would try to exercise enough to burn it off. Maybe both. Once I felt like I did enough to make up for it I was usually starving again and the binge cycle would continue. Evidently, the starving began to outweigh the bingeing because I began to drop weight and was labeled as anorexic by my family doctor, Dr. Bley in Fredericksburg.

There is so much shame and guilt that goes on with an eating disorder. My mother and step father slapped Bible verses on it like that was going to fix it. I do remember asking myself, "Why isn't God helping me?" I was in the Word extensively. My mom and step dad told me the eating disorder was sin in my life which caused more shame and guilt because I was trying so hard to stop. I had been so sheltered that I didn't even know what an eating disorder was. I certainly didn't know that there was professional help out there but that is what I desperately needed. Unfortunately, they did not get me professional help. I tried to hide my eating disorder from everyone because I was ashamed of it. My mother and step father called on the elders of the church to pray over me, which I appreciated but there was no difference as far as the thoughts and struggle. Then my parents told me that maybe if I confessed the sin in my life the eating disorder would go away, so I racked my brain and tried to think of every single sin I could possibly confess to them and, of course, there was no change. Can you imagine the damage that that does?

When I was underweight, my mother used to look me up and down with eyes of judgment and disgust. I needed her support more than anything during this time. I just wanted to feel normal and accepted. But instead I felt like an outcast.

In college I would get around eating by staying on campus all day. I wouldn't go home for meals and I would throw away any food that I packed. I would go to aerobics classes that they held on campus even with no nutrition or fuel in my body all day.

You may be wondering where my dad and step mom fit into the eating disorder. To be honest we have never spoken about it. When it first started I was so overcome by shame that I tried to hide it, from everyone, including them. After a trip to Disney with my step mom, Dad and sister and brother on that side, I remember my dad called my mom and asked her what was going on with me. I don't know anything about how that conversation went or what was said, but my dad and I still never spoke about it. My step mom alluded once to me having "body image issues." I'm sure they saw my weight fluctuate even into adulthood and throughout the rest of my life but we just never talked about it.

On the Disney World trip, I resided to eating only an apple and a few crackers each day except for one. I remember the one day because I allowed myself to have a veggie burger at a restaurant that we went to. My stepmom made the comment, "That's the most I've seen you eat all week." It certainly was. I don't know how I made it through weeks like that, especially with all the walking we did other than the thoughts are so powerful that they give you the energy, strength and stamina. Now that I have the Lexapro in me and the thoughts are so slight, I don't believe I could ever do it. I don't believe that I have the energy, strength and stamina. It's all wrapped up in the power of the thoughts.

Struggling with an eating disorder made me a completely different person. All of my time and energy went into protecting my disorder. The eating disorder changed me. I became more rigid and less flexible. I became more inwardly focused. The only thing that mattered was the eating disorder and protecting it. I remember thinking I was no longer the real me but I didn't know how to get the real me back.

I felt like I was a "good" person if I didn't eat and I was "bad" if I did eat. I started making up food rules that I had to follow if I wanted to feel good about myself and if I broke them I felt like I was a complete and utter failure. The rules had to do with what I was allowed to eat and what I wasn't allowed to eat, as well as how much I was allowed to eat. I was so preoccupied with it. Again, I didn't do any of this on purpose. I didn't know what was happening to me. I didn't choose any of this. It's like the thoughts just took over. That's why my mother and step father saying it was sin was so hurtful. I wasn't trying to do it, all of the thoughts were overwhelming. Trust me, I wouldn't choose this for anyone ever! I constantly felt fat and even though I was losing weight it was never enough and there was such an intense fear of gaining. For someone battling anorexia, no matter how much you lose, it's never enough. In fact the more you lose the more the brain wants to lose. The more you lose, the more intense the thoughts get. Even when you are skin and bones you feel fat.

My weight got dangerously low but there was SO much fear of bingeing and bingeing was the worst because it made me feel so fat and when I felt fat I felt like I was a failure and not good enough and not special. I know that sounds weird but those are some of the thoughts that were at the root. Even when I was at a very low weight I felt like I was a normal size.

This was all going on during college and it's amazing with what I know now about how an eating disorder affects the brain that I was able to keep up with my studies. I remember being SO tired at times and SO hungry when I was studying but it wasn't worth it to me to eat because it wasn't worth all the feelings of guilt and shame that came with eating. I'd rather deal with the hunger pains.

These years were some of the loneliest years of my life. It felt like I was going through life in a daze just focused on doing my eating disorder perfectly. It felt good to win at the eating disorder. It felt good to be good at something. I had lost the love of my life at the time and I was struggling with this eating disorder that I didn't know how to fix. My close-knit group of friends from high school had moved away to other colleges and I hadn't really formed any close friends at college yet because I was a commuter. My heart was still broken and I didn't know how to get it to heal.

Eventually, I came across a note card on my stepdad's desk that had a meal plan on it and other things like, "no exercising." I knew it was for me and I freaked out and had a full on melt down. I confronted him and my mom and they confirmed that they wanted me to follow this meal plan and stop all exercising. I had been running or doing aerobics on a daily basis. I didn't think that I could do this but again we were taught that if we didn't obey the authority figure that we would be "giving the Devil ground in our lives." I was still under this control even in college and early adulthood. So, I felt like I had to. The meal plan had me drinking two Ensure Plus drinks per day and eating three meals per day that my stepdad picked out. My brain was freaking out! I don't know how I got through this time of weight restoration but I did. However, it didn't take care of the root problem. My brain was still a mess. I was still plagued with the eating disorder thoughts and rules and believing I was fat. I was still flooded with feelings of guilt and shame. Weight restoration didn't automatically get rid of the eating disorder.

My parents were still a part of ATI and we went to their ATI conferences in Knoxville, Tenn., where all the girls were required to wear white blouses and blue skirts. The men blue pants and white shirts. There was a man there who was known to cast out demons or something like that, so they took me to him to hopefully fix the eating disorder. Again, ingraining in me that the eating disorder was some sort of sin and/or demon...I guess? I don't know...crazy.

My family doctor referred me to a nutritionist in his office, Jean Hoppe, in Fredericksburg. Unfortunately, she was used to seeing people who were overweight and she taught me how to count calories. Never teach an eating disorder patient how to count calories. It simply becomes one of their rules. I continued to see her because I didn't know what else to do, I needed someone to talk to and I didn't know of any other professional help in the area. Google wasn't around back then! I also didn't know at the time that it was not good to be counting calories. I was just searching for support. I needed someone to talk to who wasn't telling me it was sin or something to be ashamed of.

My mother and stepfather left me on my own when my weight was up. The meal plan they had me on had me up to a higher weight than I had ever been in my life, which was so scary and triggering. They weren't there to help at all. They were always only concerned with whether my weight was up at a normal weight. They never helped with the root problem. They never helped me seek help for the real issue. They just told me it was sin. I guess it wasn't sin anymore once my weight was stable but the plaguing thoughts were still there?

The next time my weight dropped was at an ATI event that my parents wanted me to go to. This was immediately after college and Matt and I were engaged. They wanted me to attend before we got married. You read that right. It was eight weeks in Texas with no communication with friends or Matt. Once again, I felt obligated to obey, or else, you know by now what that would mean. I literally felt like I did not have a choice. Don't get me wrong. It was actually a really great program and I have some very special friends who came out of that. But that's not the point. It's one more thing that they controlled and it wasn't my decision. Anyway, leading up to leaving I was bingeing again, probably out of stress of leaving my fiancé and my teaching job for eight weeks. Once there I promised myself I would lose the weight that I wanted to. It took awhile to get that control back but I did. I dropped some weight and I felt like I was "good" again. Like I was in control again.

I had told Matt about the eating disorder at this point but he had no idea what he was in for. When I got home from my Texas conference I slowly put the weight back on just from being back in normal life and I was happy with my weight for our wedding. My weight stayed stable for several years and although I still had a lot of the eating disorder thoughts it wasn't triggered again until I tried to lose the baby weight after our first child was born in 2003. A lot of the baby weight came off fast but that last 6 lbs. was really hard. I think I got kind of disgusted with it and then just stopped eating enough. My weight went down to my "normal low" without me even realizing it. I was shocked when I got on the scale. Matt wanted me to start eating more and drinking some Ensures (he was "enlightened about these from my mother and step father) but the eating disorder mindset was too strong by then. The lower your weight the stronger the eating disorder mindset gets. I had to do it on my own time table. That doesn't mean it was easy. The eating disorder tells you are a failure and not worthy if you gain weight. It tells you are not good enough and horrible and fat and ugly and gross and the worst person out there who is undeserving of anything good. But I had the motivations of my baby.

There were times that I knew in my head that I was too skinny but I pushed it out of my head really fast because all of the fear and shame and guilt and feelings of being a failure and unworthy and not good enough that came with gaining weight weren't worth it. The feeling of being fat wasn't worth it. So, I just kept going with the eating disroder telling myself I was fine. I mean I felt fine.

We had four kids in five years and that was a nightmare for the eating disorder. Each time I would gain enough to get pregnant and then go too far when losing the baby weight. My weight would stay too low for a while and then I would force myself to gain the weight back, mostly because I wanted to take care of myself so that I could be a good mom to my kids. I had that motivation now. Then I would get pregnant again. This cycle continued until after our fourth was born. When she was 8 months old, my health spiraled downward and my whole world changed forever.

We did initially have a bit of trouble conceiving. I hadn't been having regular cycle for years before we got married. We didn't know what that would mean. Thankfully, my OB/GYN at the time, Dr. Anderson, in Fredericksburg, put me on Clomid and it worked immediately for our first pregnancy. After that it was easy shmeasy.

It was hard for Matt to see my weight drop so low over and over again. It caused him anxiety and he couldn't focus on work at times. He sought out professional help for me and found a counselor in New York who had gone through an eating disorder herself and was now helping others. Being long d stance was not ideal but she agreed to help me via email and phone calls. I agreed as I knew I needed some sort of help and I didn't want to keep living like this. I had always wanted freedom. I remember my mom and stepdad trying to talk to Matt behind my back telling him how to handle me with the eating disorder. Like they knew how. Like they had helped me so much! It angered me when they tried to talk to Matt behind my back because it brought back all the hurt of when they told me it was sin and when they judged me instead of supported me. Again, the eating disorder was not my fault. I didn't ask for it. I wasn't doing it on purpose. I didn't need my mother and step father judging me. I needed their support. It wasn't there.

An eating disorder takes over your life. You think you have control over it but it really controls you. Everything revolves around the eating disorder. What am I allowed to eat? What time am I allowed to eat? Was I good today? Was I bad today? Do I need to make up for being bad today, tomorrow? The fear is so great that it can keep you from eating out socially with friends. It can keep you from traveling because of the new and different foods and having to stick to your schedule. It hurts you physically but gaining weight isn't worth the guilt, shame, or feeling fat. There is so much fear with eating that it keeps you friends with the eating disorder. There is life on the other side but it's too hard to break through all the fear, guilt and shame to see it. I never dealt with bulimia or self-harm but many people who struggle with an eating disorder also face these aspects as well.

Getting on the scale would either make or break my day. Should I do it? It's so scary...will I be the right number? More importantly, will I be a good number? I remove all my clothes. I don't want any extra weight. I can only weigh myself on a day that I go to the bathroom really well. It has to be in the morning before any food or liquids. It has to be the right time of month, too...not too soon after my period or too soon before or I may be carrying a little extra weight from that. I make sure all the timing is right. I step on the scale with my eyes closed. I'm scared to look. I hold my breath. I slowly exhale, then open one eye and peer down.

First case scenario: It's a low number. Sigh of relief! It's a wonderful day! I am good enough! I am a good and successful person! I can make it through the day! This is going to be a good day! I can do it!

Second scenario; It's a higher number than my normal weight, or even a higher number than I want it to be or than I expected. Crap! I suck! I HATE this day! This day sucks! I am a failure! This whole day is ruined! I can't even face this stupid sucky day! I am so fat and ugly! I can't do anything right. I can't even eat right because look at me! I am so fat and disgusting! I don't deserve to eat today. I'm not going to eat today. I can't go to work today. I can't do this. I am so depressed. UGH! I hate this. I am such a failure! I plop on the bed.

The eating disorder also tells you that you are fine. You could be skin and bones and the eating disorder tells you that you are OK. That nothing bad is going to actually happen to you. You may have a swift thought go through your brain that thinks maybe you aren't fine but you quickly push it away because the fear of having to do what you might have to do in order to actually be fine (gain weight) is WAY too scary so you won't even entertain the idea that you aren't fine and you just keep on going. But mostly you really believe that you are fine. Usually when you are at a dangerously low weight you think you are at a normal weight or maybe even a little overweight.

I began to work with the counselor in New York and she had me work though these charts that got to the lies of the eating disorder and counteracting them with God's Truth. It actually really helped calm me down, especially when I was in the middle of an eating disorder freak out. It helped me see what the eating disorder was leading me to believe and what I actually wanted out of life and thus what action was going to help get me there. For example, if I continued to follow the eating disorder's rules was that really going to give me the life that I wanted? No. The eating disorder steals your life away. We just can't see that when we are deeply in the eating disorder mindset. Nothing matters but the eating disorder when we are living in the eating disorder mindset.

Uprooting Idolatrous Patterns

Date: Time:

TRIGGERS	DESIRE/TEMPTATION What Do I want so badly to disobey God to get it?	MY PLAN How did I React Temporally or Eternally?	REALITY CHECK	GOD'S PLAN Eternal Satisfaction)
Life Circumstances Triggering the Event:	What Do I Desire - both on the <u>Surface</u> and in my <u>Heart</u>?		How Do I Feel Now?	God's Thoughts Abou Me:
Thoughts and Emotions Involved in My Response:	What Are The **Perceived** Benefits of my Sin?		What Am I Thinking Now?	God's Desires For M
My Behavioral Response to the Circumstances:	What Am I Doing? (Moving Away From, or Fulfilling My Desire)		What Am I Doing Now?	My Choices in GOD'S will:

She had me break my eating disorder rules like stop weighing myself, stop measuring my food, stop eating at certain times and, of course, adding in food. This was a nightmare. I remember crying over not measuring my milk that went in my cereal. At one point, couldn't even do it. I threw it out. I had to constantly remind myself that it was OK to eat a piece of pizza. That I wasn't going to get fat over one piece of pizza. I would freak out if there was unexpected food. This was a process. It wasn't like oh, that's all I do, OK, sure. It took time and work and effort to break my rules. It took tears and remembering that ultimately, I wanted my life back. It took doing chart after chart after chart to remind myself of the Truth. We made some good progress but the eating disorder was strong and I became pregnant with my fourth child and I needed to focus on eating for the pregnancy without rocking the boat too much. At this time, I didn't know that no matter how much counseling I did, what I really needed was medication, particularly Lexapro. That would come in the future.

My mom and stepdad had always poo-poœd psychiatric help and had even said depression wasn't real, so I had grown up with that mindset. And that was probably why they didn't get me the help that I needed in the past.

In 2009, my youngest was 8 months old and I had gum surgery. The surgery was another trigger for weight loss. The thought of not being able to eat my normal foods freaked me out, so I started getting stricter with my food intake even before the surgery. I lost a few pounds and I remember my mom looking me up and down with her judgy eyes, and making a comment about my body.

The surgery also made it hard to eat but that didn't bother me! I continued to lose weight through the three surgeries. My health spiraled downward and everything was out of control, so the eating disorder was the one thing I could control. As my health got worse, my weight got lower. There was a time it got so low that Dr. Z wouldn't even treat me for a time until I got my weight back up.

An eating disorder puts a lot of strain on a marriage. Matt was extremely worried about me. At one point, he began to push hard for even in-patient care. Every time he challenged the eating disorder all hell would break loose. Not only did try to protect the eating disorder but because my mother and step father were so controlling growing up, I would freak out if I felt anyone trying to tell me what to do in the least bit. So, it was a combination of the two. We began to argue a lot, mostly over the eating disorder and him wanting me to get my weight up. Thankfully, my Uncle Tom stepped in and was a mediator between us. It was very helpful to have that third party, someone who loved us both and wanted the best for us.

Part of me knew that I needed to go to an in-patient facility because the eating disorder was stronger than it had ever been but the idea scared me beyond belief. How could I leave my kids? How could I give up control of running the household? How could I give up control of what I ate and when I ate and how could I have someone else in control of my weight? I just couldn't do it. So, I began searching for help in our area, something that would satisfy Matt. I found a counselor in Fredericksburg who was experienced with eating disorders, as well as a psychiatrist in Richmond who worked with eating disorder patients. I didn't really know if it would help, but at the time I just wanted to shut up Matt and let him know I was doing something.

I'm not so sure the counselor did a whole lot but at least I could tell Matt that I was going. But thank God for the psychiatrist (Dr. Spanier) who put me on Lexapro right away. That was exactly what I needed. He said that Lexapro was used in eating disorder patients to help slow down the thought patterns. That is exactly what it did for me. It slowed down the thought patterns enough for me to be able to manage the eating disorder. That's how I can explain it. It's not like the thoughts are gone completely but I can tell them NO when they creep in and I can live by the true thoughts. It's not like it won't always be cool to be thin or lose weight but I have been at a stable, normal weight for me since being on Lexapro and I can live a normal and social life. I can eat in social settings and not freak out, I rarely weigh myself and the number doesn't rule my day. I was able to give up exercising. For so many years there was a voice telling me I HAD to exercise no matter what or I would get fat. I can't tell you how hard it is to live with the voices and thoughts with that kind of pressure. No matter what kind of life was happening I HAD to make that exercise happen. I'm so thankful that I can live in so much more freedom now. Of course, I know all the calories and carbs in most foods from my worst eating disorder days. All that doesn't go away but the difference now is that I can live in more freedom. On days when I feel fat I can speak the truth to myself and push those eating disorder thoughts out of my head instead of living in them as a reality if that makes sense. I have little hiccups here and there like the other day I wouldn't eat a bagel instead of a slice of bread with breakfast because the bagel had more calories than the bread but then another night I could sit and eat an entire box of chocolates without any guilt. I never could have done that in the past. It would have had so much guilt it would have set me back a week of starvation.

In 2018, I had to eat all my meals and snacks in an eating disorder center in Durham, N.C., with one of my children who was in treatment. That means that my meals were enormous compared to what I usually ate because they had to match the other patients' meals in proportions and exchanges (starch, vegetables, protein, fat, etc.) I also didn't get to choose what I was going to eat. What was served was what I had to eat. This is not fun for someone who gets comfort from being in control of what they eat and how much. But I was doing this and pushing through because it was helping my child. I gained about 4 lbs. during this time and the thoughts were strong. "You are fat. You aren't good enough. You suck. You should restrict." But I firmly believed I was past all that restricting. I had gone through so many years of starving myself. I never wanted to do that again. I hated being hungry. That was the worst feeling ever. So, I waited it out. And my body did naturally go back to its normal weight. That is a HUGE deal for someone recovering from an eating disorder.

A few months later, spring 2019, I thought I noticed that my face was a bit thin. I always notice it in my face. I stepped on the scale (I rarely weigh myself anymore) and I was down 2 lbs. from my normal. Nice, I thought. It's always cool to be a "good" number. That will never go away. Even normal people would like to be down 2 lbs., right? Should I do anything about it? Nah...it's only 2 lbs. I can fluctuate. Another month or two went by and I posted a picture on FB. My BFF said, whoa, you are too thin. I saw it, too. Crap. I don't want to deal with this! I got on the scale when we got back into town from our vacay. Down 7 lbs. total (an additional 5 lbs. after the 2). Ugh. Now I knew I had to gain. I didn't try to lose. But now I had to gain. That was scary. It's not that I wanted to be too thin. I didn't WANT to look bad. I knew when I was too thin I looked bad and unhealthy. That's not the goal. I want to look healthy and be healthy but gaining is too scary. ALL of my mind says to ignore it and that I'm fine. That's what the eating disorder does, tells you are fine. I ignored it the first day. The second day I mustered up the strength to eat extra. But the guilt PILED on. Then I was mad at myself because wasn't I past this? Wasn't I free? I had been free for so long. I hadn't relapsed in so long. And I WON'T relapse! I won't lose anymore. I won't go back! But the guilt was SO strong. I hated eating extra...and it was only 200 extra calories that day but it felt like 2,000 extra calories. I felt like a bad person. The rest of the week I went back to my normal eating plan. I was fine, right? I didn't' need to eat extra. I would wait until the end of the week and weigh myself again to make SURE I had to gain weight. That's what I'd do. I ended up eating extra only one or two more days that week.

At the end of the week I weighed myself again, but not without a TON of anxiety. Anxiety over what I ate and drank the night before because that would contribute to what I weighed the next day. I didn't want to weigh too much because that would freak me out. I knew I needed to gain weight but part of me wanted to be low again so that I had to freedom to eat more even though it's really hard to eat more. It's all a mess in the eating disorder brain. I was so scared to weigh myself that morning. Did I go to the bathroom enough, did I drink too much? Would that make me weigh more than I really am? I finally did it because I was thirsty and I had to weigh myself before I drank anything. I was 1 lb. up from last week. Crap. I started to analyze. Why was I 1 lb. up when I didn't even eat that much extra this week? Was I really 1 lb. up or was it just because I didn't go to the bathroom as well? Or am I going to start gaining when I didn't even eat that much this week? Maybe I don't have to eat extra. Maybe I'm just going to gain on my own...I knew I still needed to gain more but I was letting the eating disorder mindset take over. Then I was mad at myself for letting it run my brain. Stupid eating disorder. No eating disorder. I'm fine. I know I need to gain more. I'm going to move on with my day and I know I have to keep eating extra. Ugh.

I let a few weeks go by. I really didn't want to eat extra but I was hungry and I knew my body needed it. I wanted to weigh myself ONE more time to make sure I really HAD to eat extra. To make sure I was still at a low weight and my body hadn't betrayed me and gained the weight back on its own. I had gotten safe in my rules again, eating mostly the same thing every day at the same time and if I had to eat more it was going to be scary. I weighed myself the next week. Up 3 lbs. What? I knew I had eaten extra but it's always hard seeing the scale go up. It felt like my body had betrayed me. I kept having to tell myself, "I'm not fat. I'm not fat. I'm not fat." I continued to listen to my body and give it nutrition but not without fear and guilt. Not as much as in the past without the Lexapro but it's still there.

I share this with you because even after SO many years of a stable weight and even after all these years of so much freedom and all these years on the Lexapro I have to be SO careful. And I have to fight. I have to fight every day to keep the eating disorder at bay and keep myself safe. So, I muster up all that I have in me and tell the eating disorder, "NO! You will not take my life. I will get back to a healthy weight once again and I am in control, not you!"

I don't know what good came out of me having an eating disorder other than I could understand when one of our children started struggling with one. At least I could lend an understanding ear and I knew to get them professional help right away. It was not an easy road and every eating disorder has its own individual factors. She was in and out of treatment centers and a children's hospital for a good year and there is a high chance for relapse as I knew from my own experience.

If you are struggling with an eating disorder I have a few thoughts for you. First of all, if you haven't gotten professional help, please do. Secondly, you must stand up to your eating disorder. If your eating disorder seems to be in control right now, and you feel like you can't stop the cyclical thoughts, it doesn't have to be like that. You can stand up to your eating disorder. The only way I have learned to fight the eating disorder is to counteract all those lies, all those voices, all those thoughts that run rampant...with the TRUTH. It's a hard battle but you can win it. And until you start fighting, the eating disorder will remain a deceptively safe place. It's important that I note here that I wasn't able to successfully win this thought battle until I was on the Lexapro. The Lexapro slowed down the thoughts enough so that I could win. Before the Lexapro I was fighting the fight but the thoughts were SO strong I felt I was failing all the time. So, again, please do get with a professional that can seek out the right medication for you.

Thirdly, You can be free of anorexia forever. Freedom looks different for everyone. But I believe freedom exists. I've experienced it myself. I don't pretend that the number on the scale doesn't affect me, but I can move on from it and get on with my life even if I don't like it. I don't pretend to not know the calories in everything I eat, but it doesn't dictate what I eat. I don't pretend not to know what time I eat or what I eat but it doesn't rule me. I don't pretend not to get anxious at social events where I have to eat, but I am able to do it. I am a functioning human being who maintains a healthy weight. I can be in social gatherings where there is food. I can eat out with friends. I can enjoy food. I don't restrict. I don't feel the need to exercise. These are huge accomplishments and I enjoy the freedom. Again, freedom looks different for everyone and there are people who experience even more freedom than I have and those who have

150

not experienced as much as I have but the important piece is that there IS freedom.

Fourthly, you are more than your eating disorder. You are not your eating disorder. I know you cling to it for protection, but never let your eating disorder become your identity. It is separate from you and you need to fight it. Your eating disorder can easily become your world, and it's only when you see it for what it is--a deceitful lie--that you will be free to pursue the dreams and life that God has for you. I believe you have been called to do something mighty in your life. You are more than your eating disorder. You must believe that and fight to live your life apart from your eating disorder to experience the freedom that can be yours.

Lastly, you are not crazy. I know you feel like you are. All of those voices warring in your head. It's draining. I know you're so tired of hearing them. So tired, you sometimes believe it would just be easier if life could be over. I've been there before. I remember walking in my neighborhood in college thinking, "It would be easier if I just wasn't alive." It does get that bad. Even worse for some than it was for me. I know that many with eating disorder's deal with self-harm and suicidal thoughts. Please don't give up. You just need that taste of life again apart from the eating disorder. You need to see your life again with worth and meaning. Please remember the rest of your life is not determined by this moment. I know it feels like this is it but it doesn't have to be that way. You have an amazing life ahead of you. A life filled with freedom, meaning and purpose apart from the eating disorder. This is just part of your journey. It doesn't define you.

Like I said, It hasn't all gone away for me. I can't not think about how my clothes fit every time I put them on. But I can move forward and enjoy my body and enjoy social situations with food. I'm happy with my body now and I don't hate it anymore and for that I am thankful.

This is a far way from crying over adding mustard to my food because it would add five calories. Or crying over not measuring the milk that went into my cereal. Is this as good as it's going to get? Maybe, and I am fine with that because I am a functioning adult not ruled by my eating disorder anymore. If it gets even better, I won't complain.

Am I very aware that I could relapse at any time? Oh, yes. I don't put myself above that, not ever. Anyone who has ever suffered from an eating disorder has to constantly protect themselves.

Chapter 11: Friends during a Chronic Illness

When you have a chronic illness, you find out who your real friends are. It's those who stick around through it. When you have a chronic illness, your friend circle diminishes quickly. At least for me it did. It's not really their fault. It just happens because you can't participate in life anymore. Their life goes on and yours doesn't. Your life gets consumed with just getting through the day. I used to like going out and socializing. But that stopped. When I tried to go out I put on a fake smile and tried so hard to enjoy life but soon it was too hard to fake it. When I got home I pulled off my outfit and got back into bed and wondered if all the fakeness was really worth it. Even if I was having a "good" night, the whole evening was taken up by being scared of when the next bout would come on. How can you feel so bad when you look so good? That's a common question that I would get. Often times I would look perfectly healthy on the outside with no sign of the pain I was in.

Most people eventually stopped asking how things were going. They no longer knew what to say and who could blame them. To be honest, I got tired of trying to explain things. Most people, including extended family, simply did not understand. As Americans, we are used to a quick fix. People didn't understand why I wasn't just getting better. Many people, including the elders of the church we were going to at the time, questioned the doctors I was seeing and the tests that I was having done. I can't blame them. It wasn't their journey. And it was hard to explain and hard to understand. But I knew I was on the right track and I was determined to get better for my family. I'm sure people also questioned because a lot of my chronic pain and illness didn't show on the outside. When I went out I still showered, got dressed, put on makeup, and put on a smile. Underneath I could have very well been dealing with an explosive headache and all I wanted to do was crawl into bed and sleep for the next several days.

People are used to someone who gets sick and then recovers quickly or has surgery and then they heal. They aren't used to a sickness that goes on and on and on where there are no real answers. In the beginning, I was very open about what was going on and treatments I was pursuing. But as time went on and especially when I started pursuing a more alternative route I sensed people were questioning my choices and it just wasn't worth trying to justify myself. I had enough going on.

I was so thankful for some friends God put in my path who could identify what I was going through. I think of my friends Joan and Morie...Tiffany and Trish. All of which were struggling with their own chronic illness and we shared our journeys with each other, what was helping, what wasn't, our latest doctor's appointment and prayed for one another. Trish and I clicked right away. It was like we were long lost sisters. We could talk on the phone for hours and soon were talking on the Voxer App every single day. Our conversations grew from health to parenting, marriage and just anything in life. I could trust her to give me godly advice. We went on a weekend trip together and never missed a beat. I don't think we stopped talking for a second the entire ride there, stay over, or ride home. Unfortunately, Trish moved to Florida to seek a doctor's help and things took a turn for the worse. She has been bed ridden and not able to text or talk. I have been writing her letters and grieving the loss of her daily communication.

In 2018, I lost my dear friend Katherine. She was older than I but someone I could trust and seek advice from. I also knew she would pray for me. She was always checking in on me. She passed away suddenly. I don't know what I would do without my BFF Stephanie who lets me whine and complain when I need to without judging. We share everything with one another. I can't ever break up with her because she knows too much. I have friends like Mrs. Dowell who even though I didn't see very often, she stuck with me through the thick and thin especially through prayer. We like to take walks together and even though those got sparse through my sick days, I knew she was there. God has brought new friends into my life like my friend Kristin who didn't know me when I was at my sickest but has listened to my journey and has seen me through the end and prayed for me and supported me as I continue to get better.

I struggled a lot when friends or acquaintances would tell me of a treatment that worked for them but then I would try it and felt nothing. No improvement. Why God? Why doesn't anything work for me I would wonder!? I was happy for them but really deeply hurting inside wondering how and when and if I would ever find an answer for me. What would help MY body? Why was my body so resistant to getting help? Why wouldn't something, anything just work? Even a little bit??

Now I struggle wondering why am I getting better and my friends Morie, Tiffany and Trish are still suffering? Why is God allowing them to still be in this pain? I pray hard for Trish. I miss her. Why did my biggest chunk of physical suffering only last 10 years? Now I can function again but theirs is going on for over 20. I don't know the answers. I may never know the answers. But I hurt for them. I know Morie continues to persevere like I did. I hurt for her as I know how hard it is and I admire her.

Ironically, my best friend also struggles with an eating disorder. We've been friends since middle school. She started struggling with some body and food issues in high school but I didn't know it. Neither of our eating disorders were full blown until college. The difference was she recognized hers as an eating disorder right away but I didn't. She also didn't have parents telling her it was sin so she has been very open about her eating disorder. I am not saying that made her journey any less difficult.

I wasn't open about mine until just recently. You would think having a best friend with an eating disorder would be too close for comfort. In some ways, it is but we know how to support each other. We know how to relate to each other in positive ways. Of course, the eating disorder mind set sneaks in and we have to be VERY careful not to compare ourselves to each other. We NEVER share our weight with each other. That would make it too easy to compare. The eating disorder would want us to always be skinnier than the other and that wouldn't be good. We NEVER share sizes with each other. Same thing; the eating disorder would want us to be smaller than the other. We support each other by sharing the truth with each other. I can't tell you how helpful it was when I was in the worst of the eating disorder to have someone who REALLY understood what I was going through. No one else REALLY understands unless they have gone through it. Even Matt, who has lived through it with me, still doesn't 100% get it.

Chapter 12: Homeschooling while Sick

Matt and I decided to homeschool very early on in our marriage, before I was even pregnant with our first. Looking back, at the time, I think this was another one of our "this is what we are supposed to do because my parents did it decisions." I don't really think we were necessarily thinking for ourselves back then. But overall, I still think it has its benefits and we are thinking for ourselves today as we continue to re-evaluate every year. Neither Matt nor I were homeschooled. We both grew up in public school and we both enjoyed our public-school experiences. I don't have anything against the public-school system. Teachers work their butts off. I taught at Brooke Point High School in Stafford, VA., before our oldest, Tyler, was born. My mom homeschooled my three other siblings who grew up with my mom and stepdad. I started teaching Tyler to read at 3 years old because he was my first and I had the time. Audrey learned pretty early as well and ended up skipping a grade. Connor and Karis got caught up in my illness and I was glad I just kept them on track for the most part!

I chose the Abeka curriculum for my own sanity's sake. I know some moms choose different curriculums every year or a different curriculum for each child's learning style. Umm, no. As a mom, I need to stay sane. Abeka lets the child do the next page and lets me, as the mom, not have to do tons of planning. In fact, Abeka not only has an amazing reputation AND is used in many private schools but it is SO easy to use. I never did a day of planning in my life!

I taught my kids how to do the next page so that by the time they were in middle school, or even upper elementary, they were doing almost all of their school on their own and just asking me questions. That is the way to do it.

Let's just say I am not one of those moms who is excited about curriculum and loves to homeschool. I am a mom who loves to be with my kids and knows that it is necessary to teach my kids if they are going to be homeschooled. I'd much rather be playing with them and having a good time.

We dabbled in co-ops here and there but not until they were a bit older. Early on I felt that we could get so much more done by being home and tackling it ourselves. It wasn't until we started falling behind because of my health that we started to look at co-ops to help fill in some gaps. Co-ops are really hit or miss. We tried some that were a waste of time and the kids were not thrilled about. Then we found one in King George that was great and the kids really learned a lot and it took some of the workload off of me. The key for me to finding a good co-op was that number one, the kids were being challenged and learning. Number two, I didn't want to have to prepare and teach. Some co-ops required that the moms teach a class. No, thanks. I'd rather pay money to be able to drop them off. I was looking for a co-op to help take the load off, not add more work for me. Remember this was in the middle of me feeling like crap and doctors' appointments galore.

We also tried Classical Conversations for a few years. On one hand, it was great for the kids because it hit what we were doing at home from a different angle. But once they passed the Foundations level it was too different from what we were doing at home and unless I overhauled and changed everything we were already doing, it didn't make sense to continue. So, after a few years at co-ops we decided to take a few years off and be home. It was actually nice to be home again because we decided to move from King George to Fredericksburg and we needed that time off from driving to and fro.

A lot of people ask me how to homeschoolers get enough social time. Our kids are always involved in multiple activities. Not only do they play with kids in the neighborhood but the girls are involved music, each playing multiple instruments and participate in a local orchestra. They also have participated in our church choir and bells as well as gymnastics. The boys have played soccer every spring and fall season for as long as I can remember. As mentioned above they have been involved in co-ops, as well as home school gym and we are members of our local pool. We are not hermits.

This coming year we are back to getting involved in a co-op. Tyler is about to finish an online high school program called Penn Foster so he will graduate high school at 16. However, instead of rushing right into a four-year college we are going to have him take a few classes at a local co-op while he takes a few classes at Germanna, the local community college. Audrey is more social than Tyler so she doesn't want to do the online high school program because she feels it would be too isolating. So, she will be taking all her classes at the co-op.

Our two youngest continue to be homeschooled through Abeka. We pay someone to come to the house to homeschool them since I have gone back to work full time. We plan to re-evaluate each year.

Many people have asked me how I continued to homeschool while I was so sick. I think as a mom you just do what you have to do. At least that's what I did. At least I did the best I could. There were plenty of days that I got up and started school and then had to go back to bed. There were plenty of days that I had to leave a co-op early. The kids rolled with it. They were young and that's all they knew. Of course, I had mom guilt over it and we debated at times whether we should send them to school. We decided that the co-ops were helping fill in the gaps. Nevertheless, Karis fell behind in reading but thankfully we found a great tutor that was able to catch her up in about 6 months. They were hard little workers and like I said they kept doing the next page and I would answer questions. We made it through and they are thriving today. Praise God.

Chapter 13: Walk with the Lord

I would say I grew up in a Christian home, as imperfect as it was. When the doors of the church were open, we were there. I loved the church I grew up in. It was my home. I accepted the Lord into my heart when I was 6. Mostly it was because I was afraid of going to hell, but nonetheless I believed that Jesus died for my sins and it was by His Grace alone that I was saved and because of Jesus I could have a relationship with my Father. My faith grew slowly, mostly because of church and what my parents instilled in me. I do remember a Fellowship of Christian Athletes Tennis camp I went to being a growing point for me in high school. I remember reading my Bible in high school and knowing that I wanted to marry a believer. I wanted to raise my kids to know the Lord. I knew that much. I knew it was best for me and them.

It really wasn't until college that my relationship with the Lord reached a new level. When I broke up with my boyfriend it left pain that I had never experienced before. I didn't know how to handle it other than to dive deeply into God's Word. After all, I broke up with him because I 100% believed God was telling me to. I had no other explanation. Of course, I doubted it and wanted to go back to the relationship but God brought me to a verse in Romans that said, "If you go back I will not be pleased with you, but we are not of those who shrink back and are destroyed but we are of those who believe and are saved." So, I pressed on. But I poured into my Bible like I never had before and I listened at church like I never had before and Jesus's death on the cross meant more to me than it ever had before. I devoured Christian books and I journaled how God answered prayers.

It was a confusing time because this was when the eating disorder started and I was struggling with that and wondering why God wasn't helping me overcome that. Why were my prayers regarding the eating disorder not being answered? Why couldn't I stop? Why wasn't I good enough? I remember one time crying thinking I just want to be a good mom and I can't do that with this stupid eating disorder. There were times I felt so much shame that I felt like I couldn't even pray. I cried out to God and asked, "In the name and in the blood of Jesus Christ my Savior, bind all evil influences from me." Sometimes that helped the eating disorder thoughts to calm down. I sometimes felt like I was being attacked and I knew evil couldn't be in the presence of Jesus' name.

I met Matt in college and he was a younger Christian. He didn't grow up in a Christian home. He was growing in his faith while at college. He grew quickly, and was very soon at least as mature in his faith, if not more, than I was. I admired his love for the Lord and his passion for evangelism. I respected him a lot.

When we got married both of us had a strong faith. We prayed together, read the Bible together and were on the same page with how we would raise our children.

One year into our marriage my faith was rattled. I was hurt and angry at Matt for something he did. I once again, in the pain, poured myself into God's Word but a root of bitterness grew and remained deep in my heart for a good five years. It's not like I didn't get on with life. I mean we had four kids. But if you've ever struggled with bitterness it eats away at your joy.

Thankfully, a friend gave me John Regeir's material. Now, I'm not saying that his material is magic or even for everyone, but God used it in my life, particularly one specific prayer in his material. I remember being in my bedroom, not really expecting anything but being desperate to be completely free from the deep-rooted hurt and anger. I prayed the prayer knowing that God was powerful and could do anything. God immediately gave me a verse and comforted me to my inner core. The verse was in Isaiah, "Though the mountains be shaken and the hills be removed, yet my unfailing love for you will not be shaken nor my covenant of peace be removed says the Lord who has compassion on you." Instantly, the bitterness was gone. I remember thinking, is this for real? Will it come back? I chose to walk forward in faith believing that it was gone, and I was right. It never came back. We had the most wonderful fiveish months until my health went haywire.

Again, I'm not saying that the John Regier material is some magic bullet. I'm simply saying God chose to use it in my life. And I am grateful.

My faith and walk with the Lord once again strengthened once that bitterness was gone. However, when my health was taken from me, I was angry. I prayed and I kept up some Bible reading for a while but it shook Matt and I like we had never been shaken before. I remember people saying they were in awe of me, that I was taking this so gracefully and still trusting the Lord. I quickly was honest with them and told them the truth. I am always real with people. I think that is what life is about; being real.

In the beginning, I continued to preach the Truth to myself – that God is good and His plan was good and this was His best. I always reminded my kids that. I never wanted them to doubt God's goodness because Mommy was sick. I tried to continue my Bible reading but just as daily time in God's Word is a habit, not picking up my Bible eventually became a habit as well.

I never doubted that God COULD heal me. I just doubted that He would. I questioned His plan for me. I made a lot of deals with God. If You heal me, God, I'll do...Can't I glorify You better when I'm well? He didn't think so evidently. I was battling with the Truth that I knew in my head and the reality that I saw and didn't like it or understand. I knew none of my illness had taken God by surprise. I knew God 100% had the power to heal me. For some reason, He was choosing not to. He had other plans and I knew in my heart that His plans were good. I was battling with why He seemed to answer some people's prayers but He was choosing to seem to be silent with mine. It was so easy to focus on the negative things. I was doing everything in my power to get better and yet I was remaining sick.

I knew that God was working whether I could feel it or not. I knew that this, whatever He was doing was not just about me, it was about His bigger, better and more awesome larger ultimate plan. Yet I struggled with the day to day, the pain, my little world. Being sick didn't make sense to me and yet I had to keep preaching to myself that it wasn't about me. It was about God and His plans. It wasn't about me and my little world. It wasn't about what I understood. It was about His plan and His glory. This didn't make it easy. I had to learn that He was taking care of me even though He wasn't giving me the miracle that I wanted, It didn't mean that God wasn't working. God is always working even if we don't see it. I had to learn to stop focusing on everything that was going wrong and switch my focus to the little things that were going right. God's Word says to pray without ceasing. When we stop praying, we miss out on seeing how God is working.

I was putting God in a box and telling Him how to answer my prayers. However, in His sovereign grace, He answers us with the best answer and the best solution. I may never understand why I had to get sick, but God does and that is where we trust that He is ALL good to His children. God's plan is always the best plan. Isaiah 43:2-3: "When you pass through the waters, I will be with you; and through the rivers, they shall not overwhelm you; when you walk through fire you shall not be burned, and the flame shall not consume you. For I am the Lord your God the Holy One of Israel, your Savior."

We never stopped going to church. We never stopped believing in God or the fundamental Truths. It was just a really hard time and for whatever reason, during this pain, I wasn't pouring into God's Word anymore. Even as I started to get better, it was a struggle to get back into the habit. Nevertheless, I knew the importance of my kids knowing the Lord and we continued to go to church and buy them their own Bible studies. I'm not saying this is right. I'm just saying this is what happened. Of course, I have mom guilt over all of this and I am struggling to get back into the habit of spending daily time with the Lord. This `s real life.

In all this one thing has not changed; God is still good, still sovereign, still all powerful and still in control. In writing this book I picked up *Seamless* by Angie Smith, a Bible study about understanding the Bible as one complete story. Every step is a start.

I learned something from my child suffering from an eating disorder today. During family therapy, today they were saying how the only thing that helps is reading their Bible and I realized that I felt like God didn't help me because I was looking for Him to fix it (both the eating disorder and my health struggles) instead of letting Him be my peace and joy in the midst of the suffering. My child is letting Him be their peace and joy and that's why it helps.

I lay in bed tonight and a wave of thankfulness comes over me. I'm trusting God again. I've been praying again. I'm seeing all the ways that He is taking care of me. He has been providing for me at work and protecting me from smells. I'm seeing all the ways He is taking care of my child who is struggling with an eating disorder and is in yet another treatment center. It hasn't been easy. It's been one challenge after another but instead of being angry this time, God in His grace has allowed me to see His goodness and how He is caring for us in it. I laid in bed peaceful and thankful. It had been an emotional couple of weeks. What seemed like set back after set back, tears, miscommunication among doctors, transfers between treatment centers and units, frustration etc. God continued to open my eyes to the good in it and allowed me to trust Him again. I just pray that I can trust Him even when I can't see the good in it. I still don't know what good there was in me being ill for so long, or what good there is in me still getting occasional headaches from smells other than I have developed a sympathetic heart towards those dealing with chronic pain, or any kind of pain. But it doesn't matter if I can see the good. It doesn't matter if I understand. It just matters if I trust God.

Chapter 14: Learning about Healthy Food

I grew up being taught that the only difference between organic food and inorganic was that organic was more expensive and it was stupid. We grew up with cabinets full of packaged processed foods. That was normal to me. At my dad's there was more junk food that you could eat. I loved going over there and getting my hands on all the goods. We ate frozen pizzas for lunch and donuts for breakfast. Fast food was a norm. Why wouldn't I feed my kids any differently. That's all I knew.

I grew up foolishly believing that everything on the grocery store shelf was safe. I never imagined that our government would allow our food to be covered in poisons. I guess I am really naive. I assumed that our government would be for us. Now I wonder why our government won't let us choose the type of care we want when it comes to Lyme disease and refuses to cover treatments that are helpful like ozone therapy, which is healing to our bodies and yet permits terrible living conditions for the animals that we eat and instead of finding a solution for that, they inject antibiotics and growth hormones which poisons what we eat and what we feed our children. I find it sad that the organic food is too expensive for most people to afford. However, through my journey I have found that food is the groundwork for health. It either fuels and heals the body or is a detriment to the body.

If there is one good thing that came out of my journey back to health it was learning how to give my kids a better nutritional foundation than I had. When nothing was working, I started devouring books on healthy eating as well as reading websites about nutrition and how it affects the body. I read with wide eyes and my jaw open. I had NO idea.

I learned that what you eat affects your genes for better or for worse. Your DNA actually changes based on what you eat! I learned that our produce has far less nutrition that it did just 50 years ago, so we have to eat that much more raw fruits and vegetables. I learned that the recommended number of servings of fruits and vegetables per day was 9-13! I wasn't even coming close much less getting that into my kids! I learned about hydrogenated oils and how that was in almost all packaged foods on the shelves and in fast foods. I learned how negative that was for the body. I learned about antioxidants and how they escort free radicals out of the body and how they only come from plants! I needed more plants in my body and I wasn't getting that. I read about artificial sweeteners and threw out everything that contained them including gum and mints. There is evidence showing that they could possibly throw the brain's neurotransmitters out of balance. Yes, this seems radical but I wanted to do everything I could for my struggling body and everything I could to prevent my kids' world from falling apart like mine did.

I started throwing all the processed packaged garbage out of our house. Out went the Cheerios. Out went the granola bars. You get the idea. I started making my own kefir, making my own yogurt, buying all organic produce, buying raw milk, buying all grass-fed meat, etc. Yes, it was exhausting.

The problem was that the issue wasn't only in our home. Every family gathering, we went to, every activity or party the kids were invited to, had more junk and garbage. At first, we had them refrain. This is hard for a kid. They didn't know all the "whys" behind the changes we were making like I did at first. They were young. But I wanted to be a good mom and with knowledge comes responsibility. I couldn't know what I knew without doing the best for my kids. And I didn't want them to suffer like I did. If my chronic illness had anything to do with poor nutrition then I wanted them to have the best shot at good health if I had anything to do with it!

We asked family for help. I asked my dad and stepmom if when we came to visit they could stop buying all the junk for the kids. They were understanding and said, "There's nothing wrong with trying to be healthy." I asked my mom and stepdad the same thing and told them what we were trying to do. My mom said I was torturing my kids. She ended up putting additional rules on me and and asked me judgmental questions like, "Am I allowed to give them this kind of ketchup?" or "Well, I can't feed your kids because I don't have the right kind of food." Like chicken, vegetables and fruit were something she had never heard of. Once again, I just longed for a supportive mother.

Let me explain where this change in diet was coming from. Me getting sick shook my world and if there was anything in my power I could do to prevent that happening to my kids I was going to do it. I didn't know if me getting sick had anything to do with my diet but diet was the only thing I could control. So, as I devoured books and articles on nutrition I had to do my best with the knowledge I had. We went grain free for a while because grains turn to sugar in the body and sugar causes inflammation in the body and weakens the immune system among other things. Guys, I was scared. Scared for my kids. And whether Matt's parents and my dad and stepmom understood or not, they got on board. Unfortunately, my mother and step father couldn't find it in them to support us. You may think I was crazy, too, but I, like any mom, was and am trying to find my way and do the best for my kids.

Since I have gotten better we have loosened the reins a lot, but I still have mom guilt that I'm not providing more rigid nutrition for my kids. We do follow through on our one treat a week rule. I learned this from a friend. That's right. They get one sweet treat a week. I tell them to the best of my knowledge what the week looks like as far as what will be available at different activities, family gatherings, etc. and they have to make a choice and refrain from others. Even as adults it is important to use self-control and take care of our bodies. This is helping them prepare for making mature decisions later in life. My oldest in 16 and will be driving soon. We told him that we will lift the one treat a week rule when he is driving. We are not helicopter parents. We will trust that we have taught him enough about nutrition and he will have to make his own decisions.

All moms are trying to do their best with their kids' nutrition. I think what is most important is that you are responsible with the knowledge that you have and never judge another mom for where she's at. At first I didn't know. But once I knew, I had to take action.

Chapter 15: Health Coaching

I had already studied nutrition for my own health extensively and was sharing with a lot of people I knew. But I found that I wanted the certification behind my name. I looked around and decided on Dr. Sears' Health Coaching program. I chose his program because he is a very trusted and respected doctor who has written over 40 health and parenting books.

I completed the course and passed the exam with soaring colors. Part of passing the course was hosting my own health coach class.

I had already been hosting nutrition classes before getting my certification but I didn't have the Dr. Sears' material. I liked his material because it was very easy to follow for those just starting to eat healthy and who needed something very simplistic to follow. For those looking for something more in depth, I could get there with them as well.

I am a HUGE advocate of plants. Most people know that vegetables are good for them but they may not know just HOW good for them they are. One of my favorite quotes is from *Time* magazine that said, "It's not the fruits and vegetables are good for you. It's that they are so good for you that they can save your life."

Maybe you are taking a multivitamin and you think, "Yeah, I'm good." Did you know that your multivitamin is made up of mega doses of isolated vitamins that your body wasn't made to use or even absorb? Fruits and vegetables on the other hand are made up of hundreds of thousands of these little things called phytonutrients that all work together in synergy. Our bodies were made to use and easily absorb these phytonutrients that contain health promoting properties! When you eat plants, you are getting a huge bang for your buck.

Do you remember the five-a-day campaign? Yeah, that was the recommended amount of plants when I was in high school more than 20 years ago and for some reason that number has stuck around in most of our brains. Unfortunately, that's not enough. Today the recommended amount is 9-13!! Say what? Yeah, that's tough to get even when you are trying really hard. Trust me, I know. I was doing my best and falling short every day. Why are plants so important? Because they are the only source of antioxidants.

Put simply, antioxidants protect cells against the effects of free radicals. You can think of antioxidants as the bricks that make up the wall of the immune system. They also contain important vitamins and minerals, and protect us from environmental toxins.

Free radicals are atoms or groups of atoms with an unpaired electron. Therefore, free radicals steal electrons from other atoms in healthy cells in order to make them stable again. Unfortunately, this sets off a chain reaction of free radicals. The consequence is damage of healthy cells and tissue. The end result is harm to DNA and other cells. If the immune system is weak then the body cannot protect itself and disease will occur. We are especially prone the older we get. Antioxidants, on the other hand, contain an extra electron and give that to the free radical to calm it down and escort it out of the body. Therefore, you can see why it is critical that you maintain a high level of antioxidants in your body. If you don't have enough antioxidants to combat the free radicals it can lead to cell and DNA damage from oxidative stress.

We can't avoid free radicals altogether. Free radicals are always present. They are a natural part of living. For example, breathing and exercising cause free radicals through oxidation, however they have benefits in other ways. Free radicals are also created from lack of sleep, stress, smoking and pollution to name a few more. However, you CAN eat a diet rich in antioxidants to combat those free radicals as well as take care of your body by making sure you are managing stress and getting enough sleep.

Those who have diets rich in antioxidants or take antioxidant supplements are less likely to suffer the effects of free radicals.

Phytofoods are the highest in antioxidants. The top phytofoods are bell peppers, sweet potatoes, egg plants, kale, mangoes, apricots, turmeric, radishes, onions, garlic, cinnamon, bok choy, and berries, all plant foods.

I have struggled a lot with digestive distress over the past 10 years. Bloating, abdominal pain, cramping, constipation, and diarrhea were the norm for years. You know by now that I was on multiple medications and also was dependent on hydrotherapy for years. Thankfully, that is in the past but many people today suffer with digestive distress and I feel their pain.

The GI tract is the body's largest immune organ. I'm sure you have heard that probiotics enhance the immune barrier of the gut lining. But you also need prebiotics for probiotics to feed on. You can purchase prebiotics in capsule form, for example, Saccharomyces Boulardi is a popular one. But a diet rich in fiber also serves as a source of prebiotics.

Taking care of your digestive system is a huge responsibility. Not only is it the place that breaks down our food so that our body can absorb the nutrients. But it also shapes which parts of your DNA manifest and which remain dormant as I spoke about in an earlier chapter. That's right, what we eat turns on or off our good and bad genes. In fact, today research is showing that what we eat, our diet, plays a larger role in our health than our genetics.

Every time you eat you are either feeding the good bacteria or the bad bacteria. The bad bacteria feed on sugar and unhealthy fats. The good bacteria feed on the prebiotics, or fiber, and your body reaps the benefits. Now, this is all in very simplistic terms and the body is very complex but you get the general idea.

Unfortunately, millions of Americans today suffer from constipation. If you are one of them, chances are you have tried some of the common things that can help:

1. Staying hydrated

2. Staying moving (being sedentary can contribute to constipation)

3. Abdominal massage several times per day

4. Fiber but only with adequate hydration or it will contribute to constipation

5. Using a stool or Squatty Potty to aid when using the bathroom (having your legs/knees up in a squatting position puts the body in a more natural position for having a bowel movement)

6. Flax oil or flaxseed meal are helpful aids

7. Slippery elm capsules.

8. Aloe Vera Juice

9. Getting your thyroid checked!!! Low thyroid can contribute to constipation.

10. Magnesium

11. Hydrotherapy/colonics (used short term for a cleanse)

But you know what? None of those helped me. They help a lot of people. But not me. You all know that I was dependent on colonics for years. I even tried powerful drugs to help with constipation. The one supplement that has helped me is Mag07. It's important to note here that It didn't help at first. It wasn't until I got my body in a healthier state, cleared out infections and visceral release with Dr. Fletcher that my body was able to respond as it should. Mag07 is different from magnesium as it helps to ozonate the bowels. I found that regular magnesium simply bloated me. Most importantly, listen to your body.

Colon hydrotherapy is a method of gently filling and emptying the colon with temperature controlled purified water to soften the stool and gently empty the colon of waste. The session lasts about 30-45 minutes. There are two types of hydrotherapy systems; open and closed. Although, when I received my hydrotherapy certification, I was trained on the open system, I am a fan of the closed system. Feel free to google pictures but the open system is a tub like contracture. The patient sits over it while there is a constant water flow into the colon. The patient bears down when the colon feels full. With a closed system, the device hangs on a wall while the patient lies on a medcal table. The water flows in and then is released, in and then out. There is not a constant flow and the client never bears down. I think this is gentler on the patient and the colon. The closed system to me is more sanitary and less messy. That's just me. It is best to sign up for a 12-week plan with your first three within the same week. After that, plan to do one weekly until finished. The idea is to get to the point where you see black stool being released. That is the stuff that has been in there a long time. If you get to the point where you see waste with the imprint on it that looks like leaves, you are shedding the dead lining of your colon and that is great! Remember, this is a cleanse!

It's great to have a good cleanse but the most important way to keep your body clean is to keep the garbage out in the first place. I am a huge advocate of eating whole real food and staying away from processed packaged foods. A few years ago, May 2011 to be exact, I bought a McDonald's cheeseburger with fries. No, I wasn't planning on eating it. No way. I put it in a plastic container sealed tight. Can you guess what happened? Let me first point out that real food, whole food, like fruits and vegetables and real meat would rot and smell and stink and mold. What happened to this McDonald's cheese burger? Nothing. I still have it. It doesn't smell. It's not moldy. It actually looks good. I take it out and show people every once and a while to show them that it's not real food. Now don't get me wrong. I'm not bashing McDonald's, I'm pointing out that it's been preserved because of the hydrogenated oils among other things. Unfortunately, almost ALL of the processed packaged foods and fast foods and even restaurants out there contain these hydrogenated fats.

Hydrogenated fats, or more commonly known as trans fats are very common in packaged foods as well as fast foods. That is because it gives them a longer shelf life. Trans fats are unsaturated fats plus hydrogen. The process is called hydrogenation. This process was developed in the early 1900s and the first trans, or hydrogenated fat was Crisco. Some of the effects of trans fats are low birth weight, increased blood sugar, increased LDL, lowered HDL, decreased omega 3's in the brain, and it is transferred to breast milk. The FDA says that if there is less than ½ g of trans fat per serving the label can say no trans-fat even if it is listed in the ingredients! Don't be fooled! Check your packaged foods but even more importantly stay away from packaged processed foods and eat whole foods.

Fats make up 60 percent of the brain and nerves that run in every system in the body. The average American brain is getting enough fat, but it's not getting the right kind of fat. We need more omega-3 and DHA as brain food!

Most important to brain function are the two essential fatty acids, omega 6 (linoleic) and omega 3 (alpha linolenic). Normally, our diets in America contain too much of the omega 6 fatty acids and too little of the omega 3s. Omega 3 fatty acids are found in ground flax seeds and flax seed oil, cold water fish (primarily salmon and tuna), canola oil, soybeans, walnuts, wheat germ, pumpkin seeds, and eggs. If you'd like to learn more about omega 3s, Dr. Sears actually wrote a book called The Omega

Three Effect. If you can't get enough in your diet you should consider supplementing with the Juice Plus omegas.

In addition, I try to sneak in coconut oil wherever I can. It's a little hard with the kids because they can taste it and they are picky! Coconut oil is an antimicrobial (antifungal, antibacterial, and antiviral) and it can withstand very high temperatures without going rancid so it is the best fat to cook with. It's also said to help with energy and of course it's great in helping to stabilize blood sugar. It's also excellent for hair and skin.

About two years into my health crisis I went gluten free. I worked with a doctor who said normal antibodies to gluten should be below 10. Mine were over 300. I was negative for Celiac but had a definite gluten sensitivity/intolerance. In addition to this finding, there are numerous reasons why I will never eat gluten and why I keep my kids off it as much as possible.

Although becoming gluten free did not help me feel better at the time I learned that gluten is an inflammatory food, just like dairy and sugar. I also learned that inflammation is the root of all chronic disease. I decided that I wanted to do everything I can for my body so I have stayed gluten free ever since. I also learned that gluten is EXTREMELY hard on the digestive system. Another reason I wanted to steer clear.

Someone close to me has flippantly stated, "Well, Jesus ate wheat, so I'm sure it's safe." Well, Jesus' pure wheat was a lot different from the genetically modified and highly processed wheat that we eat today. Man has done some damage and so I refrain. I don't judge those who eat gluten and/or wheat. But I have decided that this is best for my body. We do have our home gluten free but our children do eat gluten out of the home at times.

Gluten is in wheat, barley, and rye. Gluten can cause the release of an inflammatory protein called Zonulin. This protein opens up the junction in the lining of the gut and causes gaps, thus allowing particles to leak into the bloodstream where they don't belong. This causes and immune response resulting in things like food allergies and/or autoimmune activity.

Another problem with grains today, especially wheat, is that they are heavily sprayed with pesticides. Almost all of the corn (and a lot of the wheat) today is genetically modified and most of the grains today have had their bran and germ removed so just the endosperm could be used to manufacture inexpensive, white flour.

This unfortunately means that they have been stripped of almost all of their vitamins, minerals, healthy oils and fiber and are filled with chemicals. The long-term effects on human health were not considered in this process.

Simply put, we are not eating the grains that our ancestors safely and nutritionally ate. Today, gluten-containing grains (and some other grains) are not only a source of inflammation but also chronic digestive problems. Unfortunately because of this, gluten sensitivity issues have increased drastically.

We have to be very careful. If you choose to eat grains today I would choose only organic and choose WHOLE grains like millet, amaranth, and quinoa (which is actually a seed).

In addition, grains which are refined including all of your white pastas, breads, rice and anything made with white flour acts almost exactly like sugar in your body once digested and easily spike your blood sugar.

Here are a few tips for keeping your family healthy:

1. Keep a chart on the fridge and have a family challenge like who can eat the most fruit or vegetables this week. At the end of the week they get a prize (that is not necessarily food related).

2. Get the kids involved with cooking when you can. While you are cooking, explain to them why you are cooking with whole foods and fresh ingredients. This helps them understand the value of whole foods.
3. Take them grocery shopping with you and have them pick out one new vegetable to try each week. They are more likely to try it if they pick it out.
4. Make a rule that you all have to earn "screen time" by spending time outdoors—maybe even hour for hour, yikes!
5. It often takes time to acquire a taste for something so if your family doesn't like salmon, avocado, or coconut for example or some other healthy food - make it a weekly thing until you acquire the taste for it like Salmon Saturday or Smoothie Sunday
6. Start healthy family habits together. Make a list or a calendar where everyone can plan and input their activities. Hang it up on the fridge where everyone can see!
7. Have healthy snacks prepped. I prep all my meals and snacks on Sunday. I simply don't have time during the week and if I don't plan, it's easy to eat unhealthy when the hunger strikes.

Kids' Fave Soup:

Sliced organic chicken breast to feed your family

1 package pre-washed, pre chopped onion (Wegman's)

½ -1 package organic frozen corn

1 can green chiles

1-2 cans cannellini beans

 Fill crockpot with water and cook until done.

My husband is a certified coach with Dr. Berg's program. His program focuses mostly on the ketogenic diet. My husband has had a lot of success with this diet in his own life. For those who want quick results and can stick with a ketogenic diet, this is for them.

While I 100% believe in a lot of the health benefits from this diet, I also think that many people have a hard time maintaining it long term.

For those people, my health coaching would be a better option. I focus on a 10-day jump start and then Dr. Sears' Traffic Light Eating. The 10-day jump start is similar to a detox or cleanse. Traffic light eating helps you to focus on healthy eating and portion control in a simplistic way. I encourage my clients to do the 10-day shred once per month. It is very easy and doable!

If you would like access to an online six-week health coaching course please visit my YouTube Channel:

My YOU TUBE Channel:
https://www.youtube.com/channel/UC2fkW22vh4RTYWTuLDYFp UA?view_as=subscriber

Health Coach Video 1:
https://www.youtube.com/watch?v=ZeT--1OPE-0

Health Coach Video 2:
https://www.youtube.com/watch?v=jKq2g-Ohmtk

Health Coach Video 3:
https://www.youtube.com/watch?v=0rmKJuchq5I

Health Coach Video 4:
https://www.youtube.com/watch?v=3GPpi18nX2k

Health Coach Video 5:
https://www.youtube.com/watch?v=FINMszuyPjI

Health Coach Video 6:
https://www.youtube.com/watch?v=8wjMMeTZEzo

Chapter 16: Back in Therapy

I decided to go back to therapy. I haven't been in therapy since seeing Dr. Spanier (the psychiatrist) and getting on Lexapro. That was years ago. It's now June 2019. I'm not going back to therapy for the eating disorder for once in my life. Now that I feel like the eating disorder is stable and has been for a good number of years, I thought it was time to go back to therapy to get some more of my life cleaned up. I've always wanted to continue to grow as a person. I never want to stay stagnant. I need to work on the relationship with my mother. I need to heal, actually heal, from the break up that was so long ago. I need to forgive myself for not standing up for myself when I didn't know how. I need to learn how to be a good mom in this new chapter of life as a working mom. I need to know how to be a good parent to my child that is suffering with an ED now. I need to grow as a person and learn to be happy in each stage of life. I need help with the new stresses of work. And I have friends that are there for me but I felt it was time to bring in a professional. What really made me realize that I needed to bring in a professional was when I started having obsessive thoughts that just wouldn't stop. They would come and go but they were powerful. I wanted them out and gone. I didn't want them messing with my head anymore. They have gotten a bit better but they come in spurts.

Thankfully, we tackled these thoughts during my first session. Fortunately, she told me that it's normal to have these obsessive thoughts when we aren't happy with something in our life. We turn to a happier time and get focused and stuck (obsessively) on that happier time. This made perfect sense to me. That was exactly what I was doing. I have been floundering a bit with the transition from being home with my kids to working full time and it hasn't been all rainbows and roses. My mind has gone obsessively to a "happier time" in my life. Thankfully, just being open and honest with someone about these obsessive thoughts and realizing there wasn't something wrong with me really helped. It took a huge weight off my shoulders. I also left there with a new determination that each time these thoughts crept in, I would automatically counteract them with true, positive thoughts. I was really tired of dealing with them. Thankfully that determination helped too. You know that song "Let It Go" from *Frozen*? Of course, you do. Well, my girls were playing it in the car a while back and it's very climatic and there is a part that says, "I'm never going back. The past is in the past. Let it go. Let it gooooo...." So "the past is in the past" is very cliché but it hit me, the PAST...IS IN...THE PAST. Let. It. Go. The past is over and done with and in order to move forward we actually, truly have to let the past go. We can't let it run our lives any more. We have to be done with the past in order to live our best lives now. We can't let the past define us anymore. We can't hold onto the past anymore. We can't live with regrets anymore. If we do, it's holding us back. And we don't want to be held back because we have great things to do.

I also told her, during this first session, how I felt like there was this built up frustration inside over the situation we were in regarding my child that has been in a treatment center for almost a year and how the situation seemed to be getting worse instead of better. I wanted to make sure that I didn't take it out on my child. She validated again, that these were normal feelings. We talked about how I tend to just do what needs to be done and pent-up feelings inside. Yes, I do that.

My heart is heavy for my child that is in a treatment center. It's been over a year now, in and out of Children's Hospital in Washington, D.C., in and out of in-patient care...mostly in. I don't know what to do anymore. I try to be supportive and encouraging but I feel at a loss. I can't fix it. They have to choose recovery. They have to want recovery. And they don't. My mom heart is really heavy. I have gone through all the motions. I have done all the things I am supposed to do. But it's not getting better. As a mom, you are supposed to be able to help your child. But I feel at a loss. I can't fix it. It seems hopeless. Will they just stay in treatment until they are an adult? I don't want them to miss out on their childhood. I don't know what will click, or when. It's a strain on the whole family. Sometimes I can't focus. Sometimes I'm just sad. I try to distract myself and hope that something with work, some medication, or that eventually they will just get homesick enough that it will be worth it to leave the eating disorder behind. I don't know. I decided to meet up with a friend from church who was raising two children with mental illnesses. It was so helpful. I shared with her my built-up frustration and how I didn't want to take it out on my child. She said that was normal and she had experienced the same thing. I told her how that frustration sometimes blocked me from being able to do what was best for my child in the moment. That made me sad. I needed to really practice patience. She recommended some YouTube videos by Karyn Purvis. Those have helped her tremendously with her children.

In talking with her it hit me like a brick...was I frustrated because my child wasn't' like me? Because my child wasn't pushing through and determined to get better? Because my child wanted to take their sweet little time? UGH. Not everyone is the same and the way I have handled my eating disorder is no better than anyone else. The way I have struggled through my challenges in life doesn't make me better. Everyone has to struggle through their challenges their own way. Ugh, I felt so bad and sick that I was frustrated because she wasn't pushing through harder. I am the type of person who just gets things done and does what I have to do. My child isn't like that but they have to find their own way and I have to respect that and let them figure this out their way. And be patient. That is hard for me. After over a year of inpatient therapy they finally increased her Lexapro dose from 20mg to

30mg and that was the turning point for our child. We are so thankful they are home again.

The next week that I met with my therapist, we talked about my relationship with my mother. I asked her if I have truly forgiven her, which I would like to believe, or if I'm just numb to it all because I just really have no feelings over all of it anymore. One thing she said really struck me. She pointed out that just like if my mother and step father changed for the better it would have a huge positive impact on my life, the way I respond to my mother will have a huge impact on my children's lives, either for better or for worse. Huge.

During my next session, I told my therapist how I had mom guilt about going back to work and I didn't want to look back with regret and wish I had had more time with my kids. I told her how I had mom guilt about not getting my kids to Sunday school more often and not getting them into more church functions and having more Bible time with them. She said that I carry a lot of guilt from how I was raised and asked me if my kids were good people? I said yes. She asked if I would change anything about them and I said no. There was my answer. My kids are great kids. I don't have to carry the mom guilt. I have and am doing the best that I can and am giving them the best life that I can. Yes, I can try harder to have more time with them, but not out of guilt, out of wanting more time with them because I love them. And same with church. I can pray that they will want more time with the Lord out of a love for Him.

As we continued to talk she said that I need to make sure I take care of myself emotionally and explained that because I never had anyone help me heal from the breakup that I had shut myself off emotionally and decided from that point on that I would just be a doer. I was surprised at this finding but that sounded like me. When my health went in the toilet, I never questioned whether I would just do what I had to do to take care of my kids and make sure I got better. When I was put in a job with no background or training I struggled through it because that is what I had to do. When my child ended up in a treatment center, I didn't cry...I just did what a mom had to do. I'm not a crier. I am a doer. I pent it up all up inside. Interesting....

She said I reminded her of the men patients she has because I was so unemotional. That's funny because whenever we do the personality tests at work, I end up in a group of just me and a bunch of men. She said I definitely keep everything internal and people who do that often experience health problems and she worries about me (because of the health problems I experienced). She doesn't want that to happen again. So, we need to work on me being able to express some emotions. She noticed I am not really close, emotionally connected, with many people. Why is that?

Later that night, I thought about what the therapist said, about me being shut down emotionally...have I always been like that? I thought back to when I was younger. Did I keep a lot inside? I remember feeling really alone when I was younger and not really feeling a part of either family. Did I learn to keep to myself? I remember my mother telling me I wasn't affectionate when I was younger. But I remember feeling emotions when I was in "the" relationship. Did I shut off after that? I remember going a really long time in college without even smiling. I know it because I remember the first time that I laughed again. It was the best feeling ever. I laughed so hard and couldn't stop. I don't know if not smiling was because of the break up or because of the eating disorder. Probably both. Both changed me. I remember going through a period in college when I was crying all the time so I had emotions then...I had feelings for Matt...I remember the wonderful feelings of when we first got married and trusting him with all my heart. I still have feelings now just not very many. I know I keep a lot in. I'm not a crier at all. It takes a lot for me to cry.

Matt asked me last night how things were going with my therapist and I told him how she mentioned me being shut down emotionally. He said he was glad I wasn't a crier. He pointed out how when I let things out, it comes out in frustration or anger. He's right. I hold things in a lot but when it does come out, it's not pretty. He reminded me of when we were courting and how it was so hard for him to get to know me and get me to open up. He was right. I must have been shut down a lot at that point. I was probably trying to protect myself from getting hurt again. I think I eventually opened up and trusted him because we had some really good times during engagement and early marriage.

When I was thinking about it last night I all of the sudden wondered if shut down again after matt and I went through that rough patch years ago? The one where it took me years to really truly forgive and heal. Maybe even though God gave me the verse in Isiah and healed me from the deep root of bitterness, I wonder if I shut down emotionally after that. That is the point that I can remember just doing what had to be done from then on out. Whatever came my way I could handle it. I didn't need anyone. I grew an independent spirit. I could do it, whatever it was, myself. I grew detached emotionally from almost everyone. Matt is still my husband but emotionally I think I have a protective distance from almost everyone. The therapist could see that. That's the point when I decided I was OK being alone. I had been alone before, when I was younger and my parents had divorced and I couldn't figure out where I belonged. I had been alone during the eating disorder. I could do it again. Of course, really, I need Matt and I love Matt and we have wonderful times together but there is that little independence in me, that little bit that says I'm going to be OK on my own and I can do it myself. I think I'm trying to protect myself from getting hurt again. Matt was who I trusted more than anyone ever, in my whole life. And if he could hurt me, then what?

Of course I trust Matt. Do I think he would ever intentionally hurt me? No. Do I believe he loves me? Yes. He is really the best husband in the world. He takes care of me so completely and puts me first always. But no marriage is perfect.

My therapist says I have gotten good at taking care of myself physically because I never want to be sick again. But she wants me to learn how to take care of myself emotionally. Honestly, I don't even know what that means. She said, not only do I tend to focus on just getting things done but I was told what to do my whole life and thus wasn't attentive to what my needs were inside. My whole adult life I have been the type of person who likes to be busy and tackle whatever task is at hand. I think part of that is a good thing and It has its benefits like helping me persevere through the years I was sick. But I think staying busy also helps distract me from my emotions.

My therapist asked me what did I need? What did I need to be happy and what did I need to take care of myself? The truth is, I don't even know. I'm so used to just making sure I'm busy and just coping with whatever life throws at me. She said I need to get back in a Bible study and I know she is right. I need to care for myself spiritually and I need to fall back in love with my Savior. She asked me what did I want? I don't know. I never think about that. Does anyone really take the time to stop and think about that? Maybe I was never given the chance. I went from being controlled and told what to do, to being a young mother of four, to being sick for ten years. Now, that I can breathe, what do I want? What are my needs?

That night I started to think, what *do* I WANT? If I could have anything, what would I really want? I want to *FEEL* in love with my husband every day, not just feel like roommates sometimes and in love other times. I want to feel in love all the time. But I don't know how to make that happen. Matt and I go through spurts. We go through spurts of feeling really close and happy and in love and then we go through spurts of feeling like roommates, busy with the kids and just trying to get through each day. What I *WANT* is to *FEEL* happy and in love in my marriage every day. Is that possible? I don't know...I'll bring that up at my next session.

Another thing I want is to have a great relationship with each one of my kids. Sometimes I feel like I get to spend enough time with them but other times I get resentful of having to go to work every day because then I come home tired and need to decompress and then I need to go to bed because I'm exhausted. It's easier to spend time with the girls because they are more talkative and want to go out and do things. The boys not so much. They are attached to their PS4s. But then I think of all the expenses we have and they are all FOR the kids. I started to get frustrated – the two littles still need braces, my oldest starts college in one more semester, we are still paying for treatment for one of the kids, we are adding vehicles which increases car insurance (especially for the boys), Matt needs a new vehicle, I want to continue our vacations outside the U.S....I love the tropical beaches...but my therapist said not to look at the expenses as frustrations but accept them. Accept them and look at what a good job I am doing at tackling them and taking care of them with my job. Yes, I am great at taking care of problems. I am great at problem solving. That really helped me put a positive spin on it.

I also WANT work to be fulfilling. I love to have a purpose. I haven't had enough work lately. However, I can see potential for growth and the possibility for moving up into other positions. I want to take on more work and more responsibility because that is ingrained in me. My therapist cautioned to not take on too much that I am going to be stressed because when our child comes home from treatment that will also be stressful. But I think I do really well when I have a lot of responsibility. I kind of thrive when I have too much on my plate. I do really well with multi-tasking. I hate to be bored. Being bored is the worst. But again, do I avoid feeling, by being super busy? We will have to explore that more when we meet next. For now, I will have to pick up my Bible Study and Matt and I will have to get back to Care Group at church this year.

Well after all that about never crying, I teared up at therapy today. That's pretty big for me. I told my therapist how I had been really watching my emotions over the past week to observe what she said about me being emotionally shut off. Until now, I had never noticed HOW shut down I was. When Matt wanted to snuggle in the morning and hold me I just lay there and was more passionate about what I was going to do that day. Why? What was wrong with me?

Was I always like this? I wanted to FEEL close again. I told my therapist that I only get one life and I wanted to be happy. It's not like I hate my marriage. Matt loves me. I can't remember one time in our marriage that he hasn't put me first. He's bought me huge extravagant gifts. He will run out for me and get me anything on a moment's notice. He can never say no to me.

My therapist said that she thinks that I had fallen into best friend mode and Matt had become a great best friend to me. She said she has a lot of women in her office in the same situation but worse because their husbands aren't great guys like Matt. In my situation, it's not like Matt is a bad guy. It's not like I wanted out of the marriage. But is it too much to ask to want the sparks back? Is it too much to ask to want to be head over heels 18 years later like it was in the beginning? I mean sometimes I feel that way but I want it ALL the time.

I drove home with my wheels racing in my head. What was going on? I pulled into the neighborhood and Matt was shooting hoops outside. He made a lay-up to show off and then flexed his muscles and cheered for himself. I cheered for him too and cracked up at him. One thing he has always been able to do is make me laugh. I don't know what makes him so goofy. He's like a middle schooler in a man's body. A really hairy man's body. All of these feelings of love welled up inside me. I wanted to jump on him. I did.

We snuggled that night and I didn't want to let go. I do love him I thought. There ARE feelings there I confirmed to myself. Why do they come and go so frequently? Why am I SO in the mood sometimes and so not in the mood other times. Yes. I am talking about sex. I think a lot of women struggle with this and it's nothing to be ashamed of.

I told Matt I wanted the sparks back in. He laughed. He said love is a commitment and it's normal for feelings to come and go. I said that's BS and I'm sick of people saying that. I mean, yes, it's a commitment but I believe the feelings can always be there. I mean of course we are going to argue and disagree sometimes but underneath those feelings can always be there. I think I need to dig them up a little bit.

He said he thinks we get bogged down with both working, the kids soccer, music, one child in treatment, errands, and just trying to get through the day and we end up just...at least for me I get numb...I shut down.

Not only do I need us to spend time together and talk – that's for besties. I mean, I know that we take a vow when we get married but that doesn't mean that we have to live void of romance. I'm not into it when I hear, "I'm so glad I'm married to my best friend." I already have a BFF. I don't want to live with my bestie. That's for your twenties. That's for college. I don't' want to be roomies with Matt. I want sparks to fly and romance to fill the air. That is when I am the most happy. So when I feel like that is missing that is what I work to get back.

Our sex life is good but I need to have the feelings not come and go in spurts. I need them to be a constant. I haven't figured that out yet but I think we have a start. I think a HUGE part of it is trust and working with one another to please one another and not letting the little things add up. Easier said than done when you've been married for 18 years and have four kids. But that is what I always want to be working towards. But most importantly in our marriage it's wanting each other throughout the day. It's being silly and sexy with each other constantly.

I continue to be a work in progress myself. Things aren't just picture perfect because I'm so much better than I used to be. More recently, I have struggled with this feeling of just not being happy. I talked to my therapist about it but I just kept stuffing the feelings down and distracting myself with work, the kids, and my favorite TV shows. However, when my mind was allowed to wander I got this deep sense of sadness. I had only had one time before this, back in college when the eating disorder was at its worst, that I had thought, "It would just be easier if I wasn't alive." But now that thought was creeping in more and more frequently. It wasn't like I was having suicidal thoughts. I would push the thought out immediately. I felt guilty for having the thought. I mean, I had a great husband, four beautiful children, my health was on the right track...why was I having these thoughts. When I spoke to my therapist she noticed that I was having a hard time seeing good things in my life. I was focusing on all of the hard things. It was so hard for me to shift. I talked to Matt about it and when I finally verbally expressed that I was having thoughts that it would be better if I wasn't alive, all the tears came that I had been bottling up for months and months. He said, that is depression. Once I heard it out loud I knew it wasn't normal. I called my psychiatrist right away. I hadn't met with him for years, since I was coasting on 20mg of Lexapro that had helped the eating disorder. He squeezed me in in a couple of weeks. He increased my Lexapro to 25 mgs. and told me to come back in a month and a half. I watched my progress and noticed improvement. I am so thankful. I know it's not that easy for a lot of people. So many people aren't put on the right medication the first time around, or the right dosage. The most important step is to seek help.

Met with my therapist today. I had taken a few weeks off because of Matt being gone from living up north with our child who is in the day program with an eating disorder. I needed to lighten my load at home a bit. But I was going back today and I felt like I needed it. I was feeling that pit in my stomach and the heaviness in my chest. The obsessive thoughts had come back. It's like I switched the obsessive eating disorder thoughts for other obsessive thoughts over my past. I wondered if they would ever go away for good. I ached. After all I had decided to go back to therapy for one reason – to get rid of these damn thoughts and feelings and we hadn't really been working on them enough. Mostly I just ached to know that my life was what I had chosen. I was talking to a friend a few weeks ago and she said, "You can't really blame your parents now for what your life is," meaning it was so long ago. She's right. But my mind obsessively goes back to that note and how my life might have taken a huge pivot if I just would have known how to stand up for myself in so many different situations. Why do I dwell on this so much? I don't know. That's why I am in therapy and increasing the Lexapro. My therapist said it's grief. Grief over the sense of loss. Not over a relationship. Over the loss of my childhood, my adulthood, of nothing being my own, of being controlled, and then finally, when everything was out of control, resorting to the one thing that was in control – my eating disorder.

Some of you who have suffered great loss may think this is silly. But everyone suffers different kinds of loss and I ache for all of you who have suffered every and any kind of loss out there. I decided to google grief because I decided I HAVE to get over this. I have GOT to move on. This is ridiculous. I have an amazing husband, four beautiful children, a gorgeous house, a job that provides amazingly, so much of my health back, just a lot to be thankful for. Ariel, wake up! But it wasn't as simple as waking up. I needed that 5 more mg of Lexapro. I was battling depression. Interestingly, one of the things that I found while googling was that it's recommended to write down your thoughts and feelings when grieving, to get it out there and process it as well as count your blessings. At times I have wondered if I am focusing on this too much because I am in my own little world focusing on me myself and I instead of on others. If we focus on others and how to serve them, there is less time to feel sorry for ourselves. However, I did find, while doing my research that it's important while grieving to take care of ourselves physically because grief can take a toll on your physical health and even lower your immune system!! It can lead to other things like fatigue, nausea and even aches and pains. I wondered for a split second if any of my symptoms were from grief.

I read about the stages of grief – Denial, Anger, Bargaining, Depression, and Acceptance. They said you don't necessarily have to experience all of them. I don't think I experienced bargaining. That's weird. I definitely experienced anger but I'm not angry anymore. I just see it as it is what it is. It's just what happened. I think I'm in the depression phase, trying to move toward acceptance.

I googled how to deal with regret. I hate that I have regret in my life. We only get to live once. Sometimes I am driving and I think, this is my life. Am I OK with it? What would I change? Do you ever feel this way? Are you satisfied with your life? You only get one. And I'm getting older. There isn't as much time as there used to be. Do you ever feel like now that you are 40, or 50 that you can't really change your course of life? That it is what it is now? Like when I was in high school I had my whole life ahead of me. There were tons of choices, or so I thought, ahead of me. But now, I'm in the path marked out. Unless I make some radical decision, it pretty much is what it is. It's a choice to either be happy in it or not.

So, back to regret...so I did some more googling and it was actually a relief to remember that everyone makes mistakes. Yes, I made a mistake. And just like all the mistakes I can learn from it and never do it again. Moving forward I will always stand up for myself. I will always make decisions for myself. I am so thankful that I am in a marriage that my husband supports me and encourages me to be my own person with my own voice. I will never again allow anyone to make decisions for me. I'm thankful that I can learn from that mistake and stop beating myself up for it and give a different life to my kids. No one is forcing me to dwell on the way things could have been. "The only thing that keeps us stuck in lost possibilities is the refusal to focus on new ones." Tinybudda.com Life is now and that is where our focus should be. It is more beneficial to focus on what our life can be today.

I was scrolling through Facebook today and came across a few quotes that stuck out to me:

"Healing takes time. There is a reason the Lord waited 22 years to reunite Joseph and his brothers. The lessons were found in the waiting."

"She silently stepped out of the race that she never wanted to be in, found her own lane and proceeded to win."

"It's not that you're not enough to cross the finish line. It's that you haven't yet figured out how to run this particular race. Was I suddenly going to give up just because I was unsure? No way! It's only a failure when you choose not to move forward."

This last one is actually from one of Rachel Hollis' books. I can't remember which one. But I remember writing it down when I first started work. Learning so many new things was overwhelming to me and this quote helps me put things in perspective.

A few months had gone by and I realized the obsessive thoughts over my past were no longer there.

My mind was finally peaceful. I wondered why and I thought of three things. I finally felt closure over my past, I was enjoying the high of my husband again, and I had sought out the professional help that I needed once again. When I first started the Lexpro it was to stop the obsessive thought patterns of the ED. This time I realized I was struggling with obsessive thought patterns again but in a different way and also struggling with some depression. Looking back, I think the timing of the increased dose of Lexapro was key in helping me move forward.

We will have been married for 18 years in January 2020. We have had highs and we have had lows, but I can say that I am thankful we have stuck it through the lows so that we can continue to enjoy the highs.

As for closure, I finally wasn't longing to try to change things. I had accepted the way things were. I realized that I had been trying to make up for my past and once I had learned to accept and enjoy the way things were I could move on.

I wanted to see what google had to say about closure, just for the fun of it. To see if it lined up with what I experienced. Some things I could identify with and some were kind of out there. For me, acceptance was important and seeing the past as an opportunity for learning and growth. At first, it seemed too hard to accept. I had to allow myself the time that I needed to grieve the sense of loss. Once I realized I couldn't change the past (I know that seems silly, but it's true), then I could move on and enjoy what I did have.

Chapter 17: Reality

The headaches have been worse lately. Nothing like they were in the past but I find that I am popping pills almost on a daily basis to keep them at bay. Sometimes I have a lingering headache all day and it's hard to focus, hard to think. The headaches are not like the throbbing, exploding headaches of the past, but just enough to make me not feel good. Just enough to make me frustrated. Just enough to make it hard to get through the day. They often come with a wave of a sickly feeling. I don't like this because it reminds me of the past and I never want to go back there. I find that the headaches are worse the week before my period and worse the few weeks before my next round of Botox when it's wearing off. This is normal I know. They are also worse because the person I am training wears some sort of fragrance and I am in contact with her every day. Each morning I start out feeling find and then she comes into the office around 7 a.m. and BAM, headache. I pop as many pills as are safe and my body fights. I try to press on and focus as my body struggles. I finally had to say something to her because this was Every. Single. Day. She was very understanding and we are trying to find ways that work for both of us. I never want to take away someone's right to wear a fragrance but I have to be able to function at work. I find myself frustrated again that my body is so reactive to scents. That I still can't go shopping in stores with my girls. That I can't be in crowded public places like airports or church without getting a headache. I decide to look at my diet again. I've slipped out of a strict clean diet because I was so happy at how much better I had gotten and that I didn't have to eat so strictly again. But lately I have been reminded of where I have been and I never want to go back there. I know I need to do everything I can to make sure that doesn't happen. I found Dr. Rau's The Swiss Secret to Optimal Health book. He has a three-week detox diet and then a lifetime maintenance diet. It's based on eating mostly vegetables of course. I decided to try it even if it's hard.

I'm really wanting to go see Dr. Z again; however, we got some awful news. Her license got taken away by the VA Board of Physicians because of the way she is treating Lyme disease! That's right. She is helping thousands of individuals and families but since she isn't treating with three weeks of antibiotics (which helps no one) they took away her license to practice. So now as she waits for her court date, all of us patients can't be seen by her, can't get our prescriptions filled by her, etc. Thankfully there is another Lyme specialist doctor filling in for her. I will see him in a couple months while I wait to see what happens with Dr. Z. In the meantime, I wrote a letter to the judge that will hear Dr. Z's case. I wrote a letter to both congressmen and signed a petition that is going around. We can only hope and pray. This is what we have to deal with when it comes to Lyme disease. We have to search high and low for treatments that work, and doctors who are knowledgeable in Lyme risk their license. It's sad. So as I wait to see the substitute doctor I will be running out of my compounded thyroid medication. I made an appointment with my primary care doctor but I'm sure she will question the type of thyroid medication it is and will want to do blood work. She will see that my thyroid numbers are slightly higher than normal on the medication and won't understand that that is the only way that I have ever felt normal/good and that is the only medication form that my body has ever absorbed and that we have already tried Armour thyroid and levothyroxine thyroid. I assume it will be a big mess. I can't even imagine having to go weeks without my thyroid medication. And this is assuming that Dr. Z's case in Februay 2020 goes well and we can all see her again after that. What if is doesn't go well? Then what?

****

I got up this morning feeling good, head was clear. Met Matt at Sunday School. We are teaching the 5th and 6th grade class again. He drove in from Falls Church where he is staying with our child who is battling an eating disorder. This child is in the day program now. This means they get dropped off at 7 a.m. and picked up at 7 p.m. Since Matt is doing a detail at the Washington Navy Yard it made sense for him to stay up there since his work was nearby. He was going to stay at the Ronald McDonald house nearby but they did not have a room.

Thankfully, his parents don't live too far away so he has been crashing there. He is worn out by all the driving so we leave after Sunday School and head home. After he changes out of his church clothes I give him a hug and I smell the detergent from his parent's washing machine. This may be no big deal for anyone else but for me it triggers an immediate headache. He's been using fragrance free detergent of course but his clothes have been picking up the scent from the washer that has had tons of fragrant detergent in it before. I immediately move away from him. I'm sad that I can't just enjoy my husband. I've barely seen him over the past few weeks. He changes his shirt but the damage has already been done. I try to wait it out to see if it will go away but it doesn't. I get frustrated and pop a few pills. I take my olanzapine that makes me tired. I take my Naproxen and my Almotriptan. Karis asks me to take her to Party City to look for a Halloween costume. I can't even think. I hold my head in my hands, frustrated that I am still dealing with this and am still so sensitive. Yes, I say, I can do that. Stores are normally off limits for me but I know Party City is safe. I've been there before and not gotten a headache. We venture off and as I drive I am frustrated that the headaches have been more frequent lately. I am frustrated that I'm not normal. I am frustrated that I am so sensitive and that I have to live in a little bubble to be safe and that it affects my family. I know I'm so much better than I used to be and I am so glad that I can function but I am frustrated that I

201

am still dealing with this after so many years and after so many treatments and medications. We walk around Party City and don't find anything. As we walk out Karis asks to go to Old Navy next door. Her eyes brighten. I know Old Navy gives me an instant headache. But how can I say no? OK, I say. I will breathe through my mouth and hope for the best. I stress the whole time we are in there but I am thankful that I can do this with Karis and breathing through my mouth seems to do the trick this time, plus I am pumped with meds. In the past the meds wouldn't have touched the headaches. That is the difference now. We leave Old Navy and Karis asks to go to Barnes and Noble. I say sure. I am starting to feel better. I never would have been able to go out like this in the past. This is huge for me. I am enjoying this time with my baby. "We are having a girls day!!" Karis exclaims. "Yes!" I say. I love spending time with you! I am so thankful that I can do this again with my sweet baby. Do I still have headaches? Yes. It is frustrating beyond measure? Yes. But they are more manageable and I am functioning. It never used to be like that. Meds didn't touch the headaches in the past. When we got home Matt was frustrated that he caused the headache. He couldn't have helped it though. I mean, I am SO sensitive. He does everything he can to help prevent me having headaches. I mean it's hard on me but I am sure it's hard on my family. I often feel bad for my girls not being able to use good hair products because we are so limited by having to use fragrance free. I mean a huge part of being a girl is using all sorts of great products for hair and skin and nails.

****

Matt and I are learning to stay connected even through him living in northern Virginia with our child who is still in a day program. I feel happy again and I'm thankful for the adjustment in my Lexapro. I'm thankful for Dr. Spanier who knew how to care for me when I felt things weren't right. I'm thankful for Matt, who when I was afraid to write this book because I was scared it wouldn't be good enough said, "Look at it as a learning experience. Look at it as an opportunity for growth. It doesn't have to be perfect." He knows me so well. I'm thankful for his encouragement and support. I'm thankful for continued work with my therapist and that the door to my feelings is opening up again. I'm thankful for every moment that I feel in love with my husband. It will be our 18-year anniversary in January 2020. As we lay in bed this morning, we reminisced of all we had been through. It hasn't necessarily been easy but we are grateful we are together.

Chapter 18: Kids Being My Joy

I'm SO thankful I didn't get sick until after I had my kids. Of course, I cried out to God asking, "Why did you give me these precious babies and then make me sick so I couldn't even take care of them and be a good mom to them!?" But ultimately, of course, I am SO glad I have them. They are my rays of sunshine. The brightest part of my day was and is seeing my kids' faces and their delightful smiles. I don't think I would have gotten through the years of illness without their hugs, snuggles, and beautiful faces. People asked me how I did it when I was ill and you know, as a mom you just do what you have to do. It doesn't really matter how you feel. The kids were also understanding. It was just life to them. When Mommy needed to rest, Mommy needed to rest. When Mommy had a headache, mommy had a headache. When we all had to pile into the van to go to the doctor's, that was just a normal day. I longed to be a normal mom again. I wanted to do fun things with my kids without being in pain. I longed to be the mom that I pictured being. But that was not in God's plans for me. I was thankful though that I had these four precious children to get me out of bed every morning. I wonder if I didn't have them if I would have spiraled into despair. Over the years they kept me laughing. Here are a few things that I jotted down over the years that kept me laughing even in the pain.

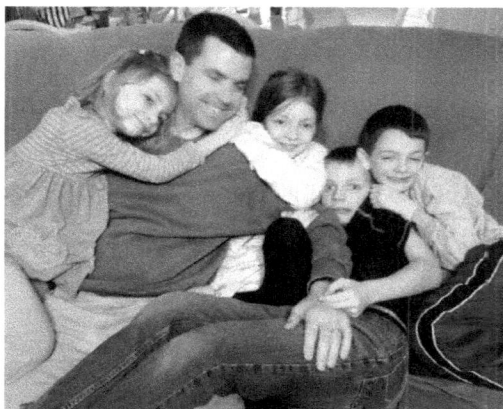

2011 Quotes

Tyler is 8, Audrey is 6, Connor 4, and Karis 3.

Ariel was REALLY tired and had her eyes closed while Audrey did her reading to her out loud…

Karis: "Mommy, why you are closing your eyes?"

Ariel: "Because I'm tired. I want to go night night."

Karis: "But we need you!"

Ariel: "You do? Why?"

Karis, thinking for a minute: "Ummm, because…we still hungry!!"

We got Netflix in January…

Audrey: "Now we don't need to go to the library anymore, we have our own little library."

Karis was chasing Connor around the house trying desperately to put her lei (Hawaiian necklace) on him…

Connor: "KARIS! Stop! I do not want that!"

Karis: "But, Connor, I want to make you fancy! It is so fancy! You can be fancy, Connor!"

Connor: "I am a BOY, Karis! Boys are not supposed to be fancy!"

Audrey: "I want an umbrella for my birthday. One with sleeping beauty on the place where I hold it."

Tyler: "Umbrellas are for girls! Boys can just get wet!"

Audrey: "Mommy, am I going to be a GOOD mommy when I grow up?"

Ariel: "Yes, of course, you will!"

Audrey: "Because I'm so good and taking care of babies and doing jobs around the house."

Karis: "Mommy, when Audrey is a mommy, what are you gonna be?"

Ariel: "I'll be the grandma."

Audrey: "And Mommy, since you've been such a good mommy to us, when I have kids, I'll talk to my husband and ask him if it's OK if our kids come to your house to sleep over."

Ariel: "Oh, I would love that!"

Audrey: "They might be shy because they won't know you very well at first."

Ariel took the girls to her sister's bridal shower. Audrey and Karis were "helping" with the gifts. During one gift opening Audrey found some underwear..."Look at this crazy underwear!! Ha ha! Mommy! Why does she want THAT kind of underwear!?"

Let's just say everyone got a good laugh at that point.

Ariel was getting gas with the kids in the car. Afterward, Tyler said: "Mommy, is THAT how much the gas costs?? FORTY dollars?"

Ariel: "Yep."

Tyler: "Gas is a waste of money!"

Ariel: "Well, it's not really a waste because we need it if we want to go anywhere, but you are right that it's expensive."

Tyler: "These gas stations must make a lot of money!" After thinking for a moment. "Maybe Daddy should work at the gas station so he can get lots of money for all the doctors!"

Karis: "Mommy, do you have some meat for me?"

Ariel: "I have some chicken."

Karis: "Mommy, I'm not a chicken girl. I'm a MEAT girl."

Ariel was on her way home from Fairfax with all the kids in the car stuck in LOTS of traffic...

Karis: "Mommy, how we gonna get home with ALL those cars in our way!?"

Driving in the car...

Connor was quizzing Karis on what the traffic light colors mean

Connor: "Karis, what does green mean?"

Karis: "Go."

Connor: "Good job, what does yellow mean?"

Karis: "Ummm...I don't know."

Connor: "That's OK, Karis, we'll do that one again since you got it wrong. Yellow means slow down. What does red mean?"

Karis: "Stop."

Connor: "Yep. Now what does yellow mean?"

Karis: "Slow down."

Connor: "Mommy, aren't I doing a good job teaching Karis!?"

Karis: "NO, Connor! I can take care of MYSELF!! You are not teaching me!"

A few days later...in the car again...

Karis: "Connor, what does green mean?"

Connor mumbles and rolls his eyes: "Go."

Karis: "Connor, what does yellow mean?"

Connor mumbling again: "Slow down."

Karis: "What does red mean?"

Connor:"KARIS! Please stop asking me questions! I am just trying to rest and have a nice peaceful ride!"

Tyler and Audrey playing outside trying to fix something...

Ariel: "What's going on? What do you need?"

Tyler: "Mommy, you don't know about this stuff, so don't worry about it. It's our pop gun and you are not a gun gir , so you don't worry about these things!"

Karis on the potty for a really long time (as always)...

Ariel: "Karis, are you done yet?"

Karis: "No, don't ask me. I will tell you when I'm done."

More time passes...

Ariel: "Karis! Are you done YET?"

Karis: "No! I will be done in 15 more minutes."

Karis: "Mommy, would you like some tea? It's gluten free tea!?"

Tyler, reading his Ben Franklin book: "Mommy, am I going to be a great man in history?"

Karis: "Connor, when I'm a grown up you can come to my house."

Connor: "Eh."

Karis: "But Connor, I will cook you some dinner and make you some cookie dough!"

Tyler: "Mommy, one day you and Daddy are going to be like Mrs. Relax and Mr. Relax because Audrey and I will be able to do everything and you can just sit around while we take care of everything."

In the car...Tyler: "I hope we have another baby one day."

Audrey: "Yeah, I hope it's twins! A boy and a girl!"

Tyler: "Yeah, and we can do everything for the babies. Mommy won't have to do anything."

Connor: "Yeah, Tyler can make the bottles, and I can bring the babies toys, and Karis can play with the babies, and Audrey can feed the babies. Mommy, you won't have to do anything, because we can do EVERYTHING for the babies. You can just rest."

Audrey: "Yeah, Mommy, you can do all the other chores in the house while we take care of the babies!"

Tyler and Audrey were doing their spelling and Matt was making up a sentence for every word. The word was "biggest."

Matt: "Biggest. Daddy has the 'biggest' muscles in the whole world! Biggest."

Audrey, in all seriousness: "No. Uncle Tom does."

Karis: "When me and Audrey are mommies, we're gonna be mommies in different families, and Tyler and Connor will be daddies in different families. So, you won't have to take care of us anymore."

Ariel: "But I love to take care of you. Can I take care of your babies?"

Karis: "If you invite us."

Ariel: "Oh, I will definitely invite you."

Karis: "Well...do you have cribs for my babies?"

Matt, trying again: "Daddy is the strongest in the WHOLE world, right, Audrey!?"

Audrey: "No, Uncle Tom and God are the strongest!" (Uncle Tom is right up there with God now!)

We were all talking, debating, etc., over whether or not to take a walk. Everyone wanted to go except Tyler and he was getting a little perturbed…

Tyler: "OK! Let's just keep this all under perspective!"

Matt was lying in Karis' bed with her at night…

Karis: "I like Daddy. And I like Mommy. And I like Tyler and Audrey and Connor…and MOSTLY I like my WHOLE SELF!"

Ariel was sweeping the floor for the millionth time that day. Audrey said: "When we all learn not to drop crumbs on the floor we should have a party!"

Ariel was folding clothes with Karis and said: "Ugh, I'm tired."

Karis: "You can take a nap."

Ariel: "I can?"

Karis: "Yeah, because we know the right and wrong choices."

Ariel: "Oh, well, I guess you do."

Karis "Because you teached and trained us."

Ariel: "Well, then, guess I'll just go lie down!"

Tyler: "Maybe when I grow up I"ll have a store with EVERYTHING you need there, Mommy. Everything will be healthy and not expensive and all at one store. Do you think I should do that?"

Matt was lying down with Karis at bedtime .

Karis: "Daddy, can you lie in my bed forever? I'll bring you toys and lunch. Can you do it?"

We were outside today and the kids were playing by the edge of the woods. Audrey was sitting up in a tree and Matt walked over and said: "Look, Audrey, watch this, I think this big branch is dead." Then he broke off a HUGE branch and held it up above his head and said: "YEAH! Look at that, Audrey, I'm stronger than Uncle Tom now, aren't I?!"

Then Audrey said: "NO. Uncle Tom can knock down trees that are still alive."

I guess he'll keep trying.

We were visiting a chiropractor's office and the waiting room has massage chairs. The kids thought this was WONDERFUL, as did I. As they were trying them out Tyler decided it was MUCH more fun to be controlling everyone's controllers than actually sitting in the chair and said: "Mommy! I LOVE controlling everyone!"

Me, too, Tyler...me, too! Like mother like son, unfortunately! Poor guy is getting all my negative qualities!

Matt was taking Audrey to the doctor's:

Tyler: "Mommy! Can I go with them?"

Ariel: "No, there's no reason for you to be exposed to more germs."

Tyler: "But Mommy! If I stay home then I'll just be bored and then I'll get in trouble."

Ariel: "Well, that's your choice. You are responsible for your actions."

212

Tyler: "I know! But I don't want to do the wrong thing or act the wrong way BY ACCIDENT!!"

2012 Quotes

Ariel was telling Karis something she wasn't too thrilled to hear. After a short pause Karis said: "I got ALL of Mommy's voices out of my head!"

Tyler: "Why can't Daddy just be like Grandad and get a check every month but not go to work?" (Grandad is retired.)

Tyler: "Why do I have to do school? I mean, don't I know enough? Can't I just go get a job and provide for my family?"

We were watching *Funniest Home Videos* together in the basement and Matt kept switching to ESPN during commercials, as he is known to do. Audrey, finally fed up with it said: "Can you please go to bed so I can take control of the remote?"

Karis: "Daddy, why don't you know ANYTHING!?"

This gave Ariel a nice laugh from the other room.

Tyler: "Mommy, wouldn't it be so nice and fun if I was the ONLY kid in our family?" (There's a big smile on his face.)

Ariel: "Well, that would be fun because I love you so much but I also love my other kids."

Tyler: "Well, I mean, I love them, too...but sometimes they can be such a pain in the back!"

Audrey: "Mommy, do you know what the BEST part about believing in Jesus is? That my favoritest most funnest day ever will be when I die and go to heaven and get to see Mary and Joseph and Gabriel and all those people!"

Connor: "Yeah, and that will be my favorite day, too because in heaven I won't cry or get consequences...it will be SO fun!"

Ariel: "Karis, come here so I can snuggle you."

Karis came over for a quick hug and then tried to get up.

Ariel: "I'm going to keep you here forever."

Karis: "No! Because I have to dance...and EAT!"

Matt: "Karis, you are such a good snuggler! Can you teach me how to snuggle?"

Karis: "Daddy! Snuggling is EASY!"

Ariel was getting ready to read Karis' blessing to her and was explaining it to her:

Karis: "But did you put that I was cute in there?"

Ariel: "Well, let's just read it."

Afterward:

Karis: "But you didn't say that I was cute!"

Ariel: "Well, we already know you are cute."

Karis: "But you might forget and I do lots of cute things!"

Karis was being argumentative...

Matt: "Karis, you need to learn that when Daddy or Mommy say "no" then you don't keep asking over and over."

Karis: "Well, you need to learn to not say no to me! Do you know who is the boss of you? GOD!"

Audrey: "Mommy, when I grow up I think I'll be a vet first before I get married. Then after I get married I'll have some kids. And you can come and visit my kids. I think I'll have four kids like you have four kids." (Her eyes got big and wide and a big smile spread across her face) "Then MY kids can play with YOUR kids!"

Karis was bothering Connor the whole way home.

Ariel: "Karis, don't say anything else to Connor about his boat or you are going to have a consequence when we get home."

Karis didn't obey.

Ariel "When we get home you will have a consequence."

Karis: "Well, you'll have to catch me!"

Ariel: "If I have to catch you then you'll have more consequences!"

Karis: "Weeelll, I like Daddy better than you!"

In the car, Karis and Connor arguing about who is older:

Karis: "Well, I'm 11 so I'm the big sister!"

Connor: "I'm 13 and 13 is a teenager and a teenager is bigger than a big sister!"

Karis: "Well, I'm 18, so I am bigger."

Connor: "Well, I'm 20teen and that's an adult! So, I am older!

Karis:Weeeellll...I'm the 50teen!"

Connor: "I'm a SOLDIER, BAM!"

Karis: "Weeellll..."

Connor: "Karis, say you're a policeman, you can be a policeman."

Karis: "I'm a police man so I'm the biggest because can put you in jail!"

Connor: "Well, I'm the sheriff, so all you are is my helper."

Karis: "OK, I can be your helper, Connor."

Connor: "Yeah, we can play that I'm the sheriff and you are the helper and we can get ALL the bad guys together!"

In the car:

Tyler: "Mommy, when we get a new van what color do you think it will be?"

Mommy: "I'm not sure, we just have to look around for a good deal and see what color it is."

Karis: "Weeelll. You can just paint it our favorite color, pink!"

We were listening to the Casting Crowns CD in the van on the way to Community Bible Study.

After singing for a while Karis said: "Me and Mark (the lead singer) are the best singers. I know all the words and sing the whole song on the CD. Even when I dance I sing all the words."

Karis was doing yoga moves in the living room

Ariel: "We have to start doing yoga again."

Karis: "Yeah, especially the balance ones. You know why I can do yoga with you? Cause look at my BIG muscles (showing me her muscles). They are REALLY BIG like your muscles, Mommy! (If that alone doesn't give you a laugh!) Mommy! That is like we are TWINS!"

Ariel: "Karis, can you tell me your Bible verses that you learned at Bible study?"

Karis: "Ummm, we have four"

Ariel: "Can you tell them to me?"

Karis: "Ummm, yeah, one is a Matt one (Matthew reference) like Daddy's name..."

Ariel: "OK, what is it?"

Karis: "And, one is a Mommy one!...HA HA, just tricking!"

Connor: "Mommy! Can we have an Easter egg hunt TODAY?"

Ariel: "Yeah, I think so."

Tyler: "Why do we have Easter egg hunts anyway? I mean what does that have to do with Easter?"

Connor:"TYLER! Egg hunts are SO fun! Don't you know the real spirit of Christmas!?"

Karis "I like being cute. It sure is fun to be cute!"

We were watching an old movie and a lady was using a pay phone.

Tyler: "Mommy! What is that? Do they have to PAY to use the phone?"

Ariel: "Yep, it's a pay phone."

Tyler: "Well, that's RIDICULOUS! Why don't they just use their cell phones?"

Karis: "Daddy, are you wondering what I'm doing?"

Matt: "No, should I be wondering what you are doing?"

Karis: "Daddy, be quiet so I can focus!"

July 4th, Karis and Connor on the fireworks:

Karis: "Wow! Connor! It's like MAGIC! Isn't it, Con?"

Connor: "Yeah, or like BULLETS, bullets all over the sky!"

Karis: "Yeah, it's like magic behind them, Con, like magic!"

Connor: "Yeah, or like bombs, bombs exploding everywhere!"

Karis: "It's magical."

Connor: "Yeah, explosions everywhere!"

In the car:

Connor: "You know, Karis I pretty much teach you everything you know."

Karis: "Wow, Con, you know a lot! Do you know EVERYTHING?"

Connor: "Yeah, I know everything... (long pause), Weeelll, I DON'T know the things when I was in Mommy's tummy, but I know everything AFTER that."

Leaving a doctor's office:

Tyler: "Gosh, Mommy, everyone kept saying how good we were."

Karis: "And everyone said how cute I was! Right, Mom? EVERYONE said I was sooo cute!"

Tyler asked: "Mommy, how do people TRY to get pregnant? Do they like eat certain foods or something? Or do they just pray and hope it happens?"

Karis: "Mom, I definitely do not want to marry a soldier because I do not want my husband to go to war and I do not want him to get dead! Then I'll have to get a new husband!" (She crosses her arms over her chest.)

What is the hardest thing you've ever done?

Connor: "This is hard, I try to not open my Christmas presents when it's not even Christmas!" (Pause.) "I know what is the hardest thing! Not to sin! That's HARD!"

Tyler: "Mommy, there is one commandment that our family doesn't obey the most – obeying your parents!"

Audrey: "Well, MOST kids have the hardest time with THAT commandment!"

2013 Quotes

Ariel: "Karis we have to leave at 9:30 tomorrow so I'm gonna wake you up at 8:30 to get ready."

Karis: "Well, wake me up at 8 because I'm always rushed because I don't do ANYTHING fast when we go somewhere."

Connor yelling for Karis from the basement to come:

Karis: "No, Con. You are just going to shoot me with a Nerf gun and I have better things to do."

Karis: "Con, whose house would you like to have the holiday's at when we are grown up?"

Connor: "Karis! I don't think we need to worry about that now!"

Karis: "Well, I'm happy to have it at my house but it's probably going to be really messy because I'm going to have lots of pets!"

Audrey: "Mom you've been a little more cranky lately."

Karis: "Audrey! That's because she has long days and we don't listen!"

Karis: "I used to think pizza was great! Then I had Bonefish and I was like, oh my gosh, pizza is disgusting!"

Karis: "Mom, we shouldn't have to ever do chores if everyone would just stop making a mess!"

Karis: "Mom, can you get me some water?"

Ariel: "Why can't you get yourself some water?"

Karis: "I'm busy...playing Kindle."

Ariel mentioned she wasn't thrilled with our plans for the evening:

Tyler: "Mom, remember we let you go to all your network meetings and meet with your friends and do your business stuff so you can do one night of this! That's what you say to us when we don't want to do something! We get to play with our friends all the time, so we can suck it up!"

Karis: "Mom, I just don't understand bad guys. I mean why can't they just make friends. I mean, Abraham Lincoln made the South be friends with the North eventually!"

Matt to Karis: "I need to have dreams like Mom."

Karis: "Mom doesn't have dreams. She has goals. She doesn't dream about it!"

Connor: "I'm SO glad I'm not a girl so I don't have to EVER give birth!"

Karis: "Well, I'm SO glad I AM a girl because when I grow up I just want to stay home and snuggle my babies ALL day!"

Tyler: "Mom doesn't just stay home!"

Connor: "Yeah! Mom works hard! She doesn't just sit around!"

Ariel: "Connor, Dad is going to get some groceries. Anything you need?"

Connor: "Yep! Steak and salmon!"

Karis: "Another reason I want to move out is so I can do whatever I want and eat Oreos!"

Karis: "Mom, what do you really want for Christmas ? I mean, you always ask for like new kitchen towels or socks and boring stuff like that. I mean, what's something that you just want that you don't ever ask for. I mean, that's what Christmas is all about...oops, I mean Christmas is about the one most important thing: Christ coming into the world as a baby!"

Tyler: "Mom, what is your most pressing issue?"

Connor: "YOU!"

Connor: "Mom! Don't come in here! Everything is FINE!"

Karis doing writing: Ugh, Mom! Can I just voice text it to you!?"

Connor: "Mom, I'm taking Leo (his pet turtle) outside so he can fulfill his dreams!"

Tyler: "Ugh, Mom, stop! I'm trying to control the conversation and I can't do that when you keep butting in!"

Ariel: "Karis, do you have any pressing issues we need to talk about?"

Karis: "Yes! I need a giant Kit Kat bar and a pet!"

2014 Quotes

According to Karis, life is terrible today because she has to clean her room. I am such a mean mommy!

Karis: "But Mommy, my stuff GOES on the floor because that is how I find it! If I clean it up I lose everything!"

Ariel: "Connor, we need to do school. Where are you and what are you doing?"

Connor: "I'm running around the house like a crazy person." (He was actually.)

Karis: "Mommy, I think I am turning into a grown up because I act like a grown up and I like grown-up shows even though you don't let me watch them."

Connor: "Mommy, look at all that snow out there! It has no one to play with it!"

Ariel: "Tyler, get focused on school, buddy."

Tyler: "I'm having a lollipop. I'm being very productive."

Karis (5 years old) while driving home from Walmart:

"Dad, why do the trees go by faster when you are driving? They seem slower when Mommy's driving."

Ariel and Connor working on language:

Ariel: "And what comes at the end of a sentence?"

Connor: "A little dot."

Ariel: "And what is the little dot called?"

Connor: "A pyramid."

Ariel: "What do you want to be when you grow up?"

Audrey: "A doctor."

Ariel: "What kind? For animals?"

Audrey: "No, for kids."

Ariel: "Oh, a pediatrician! You'd be good at that."

Audrey: "I know."

Ariel: "Well, you better keep working hard on your school stuff."

Audrey: "Yeah, I want to go to college so I can get a computer with Facebook."

Karis: "I'm bored. I wish it was my birthday because I'm never bored on my birthday!"

Tyler pondering whether or not to spend his birthday money on a new Wii game: "If I just save my money my whole life then I'll just end up spending it on college, which isn't exactly that fun, so I might as well enjoy it and take advantage of my birthday money and stuff."

Karis wanted to ride her bike this morning. I attempted to walk/jog along side her (keep in mind I haven't really exercised in a LONG time because of feeling so ill). She said, "Mommy! You are pretty fast for all your problems! I mean, headaches going to explode, and what is that other thing...oh, yeah, thyroid issues and tired." Thanks Karis!

Matt was asking the kids who wanted to go to the library. The girls jumped at the opportunity. Connor said, "Nah, I'll stay home with Mommy and give her hugs when she feels like crap."

Tyler: "Mommy if you are still sick when us kids are grown up, then I'm going to call or text the other kids and tell them to all give you money for your birthday like $3,000 each so that you can go to that center and get better."

Sigh, I have the sweetest kids!

Earlier this week Tyler was doing school and said: "Ugh, I hate when they teach me new stuff. I wish we could just do the same old easy stuff."

Connor was grumbling doing the dishwasher.

Tyler said: "Connor, your life is so easy compared to mine! I didn't even know what life was when I was your age!"

Matt took the three younger kids for a quick outing. Tyler and I are just hanging around at home and he said: "I like hanging out with just you, not all those crazy kids around!" He thinks he is the third adult in the house.

2015 Quotes

One night on our way home from our friends' house Tyler said: "Mom, did you hear her say how well behaved we were? They have NO idea!" Audrey chimes in: "Yeah, she said she hopes her kids learn from us but I hope not!"

Oh, goodness...at least they see the difference between how they act at home and out...just gotta work on the home part!

There is a bomb threat at the doctor's in D.C. and we had to evacuate the building:

Tyler: "That's stupid. I mean, if the person really wanted to blow us up why would he call and say 'Hey, I placed a bomb! Everyone get out!'"

Conner: "We get mad plenty of times and don't place a bomb!"

Learning about tycoons at the Classical Conversations Co-op:

Teacher: "What were the men that made a ton of money called in the 1800s?"

Connor: "Oh! Raccoons!"

Close, I'm thinking.

Tyler: "Being a mom is SO easy! How about we switch lives today and you can do my school and ask me questions about it and do my chores and complain about it like I do and I'll clean the bathrooms and answer everyone's school questions like you do and feed everyone and do Voxer and computer like you and I'll show you how easy it is to be a mom!"

Ariel: "Tyler, I am getting really angry at you for not focusing on school today!

Tyler: "Sorry, I have to focus. I can't talk right now."

Tyler: "I wanna go to Pop and Adee's house. I need some adult conversation."

Karis: "Mommy, what are you reading?"

Ariel: "Just a book about how to be a better mommy."

Karis: "What!? You already are the goodest mommy there is! You do school with us, you don't let us starve and I wouldn't want anyone else to snuggle me!"

Connor and Karis having a conversation this morning:

Connor: "Karis, hurry and do your school so we can play, come on!"

Karis: "I haven't been getting good sleep lately, Con."

Connor: "Well, have you been holding your blanket?"

Karis: "Yes, Connor!"

Connor: "Have you been closing your eyes?"

Karis: "I think so. I just have been getting to bed too late I think."

Problem solving at its finest!

Connor: "Karis! Pleeeaaassseee hurry up and do your school so we can play!

Karis: "Connor! Don't be the judge of me!"

Audrey: "Mom, I HATE football! It's so boring I don't know who would like it! Who would want to watch people running around tackling each other and getting hurt from trying to get a ball!?"

Connor: (knowing Audrey loves gymnastics) "Who would want to watch people swinging on bars and doing cartwheels!?"

Tyler was trying to bother Connor and be obnoxious toward him.

Tyler: "Connor, now you know how it feels to be bugged and bothered!"

Connor: "I didn't even know you were bothering me, so actually I don't know how it feels!"

Audrey: "Trust your instincts! Well, unless your instincts are terrible."

Tyler: "Mommy, how long have you and Daddy been married?"

Ariel: "Almost 14 years."

Tyler: "Wow! That's a looong time! You must be tired!"

Tyler: "I'm glad I'm not a girl so I dont have to give birth."

Tyler: "Audrey, you don't have to get me much for my birthday. Just get me some gum because I don't want you to spend a lot of money on me."

Audrey: "But it's fun to spend money, so I want to get you more."

Tyler: "No, it's not fun to spend money!"

Karis: "Well, for a lot of girls it is, Tyler, so that's why I am getting you lots of things for your birthday!"

Quote of the Day from Connor at bedtime: "Can I go back downstairs real quick to clean up something so that you and Mommy don't freak out when you see it? I'll be quick."

Audrey: "Mommy could we survive in a desert?"

Connor: "If we had Juice Plus shake!...and milk...or water...and a cup...and a spoon."

Audrey: "It takes SO long to get in and out of New Jersey because of that big pike thing." (The New Jersey Turnpike.)

Connor: "You make me so mad!"

Karis: "Stop talking! I just want you to stop talking!"

Connor: "Well, you need to behave! You don't even know how to behave!"

Karis: "That's because you make me mad!"

Connor: "I don't make you mad! You are just SO annoying!"

Karis: "I just want you to stop talking!"

Audrey: "Karis, you are being so annoying!"

Karis: "No, I'm not, you are being mean."

Audrey: "I'm just annoyed because you are so annoying to me!"

Siblings at their best. Tyler would be right in there but he's at a soccer ref training. Nothing like a cheery Sat. morning!

Tyler passed his ref class today whoo hoo! "Mom, the guy said we have to get something because I'll have to pay taxes or something."

Ariel: "Yeah, everyone with a job has to pay taxes."

Tyler: "WHAT?! That's ridiculous!! I'm like working to pay the government! Who would do that?!"

Tyler was trying to convince me to end his no Xbox consequence early:

Ariel: "Tyler, I know you are usually a good boy."

Connor interrupts: "MOMMY! Seriously! Usually!? TELL THE TRUTH!"

Matt was doing family devotions. After a long explanation of a passage Tyler looked in deep thought:

Tyler: "Dad, are the Redskins playing today? They've been doing better beating the Cowboys and other teams. It would be fun to watch if they are on today."

I think what Matt was sharing is really sinking in.

Oh, a boy after my own heart!

Connor: "Mommy! I did all the equations and they are SO fun!"

Tyler: "What equations?"

Connor: "Tyler they have letters and you have to figure out what they are and it's SO great you are gonna LOVE them! It's easy and it's fun!"

Audrey: "Ugh, everything is fun until you say no about something!"

Connor: "Sometimes I do a contest to see how long I can pinch my butt. My record is 45 seconds!"

Tyler:"Mom! You have BIG teeth!"

2016 Quotes

Matt told Karis she wasn't allowed to have something. She was upset and Tyler said: "Don't worry, Karis, Dad's not in charge...I mean, he is but not as in charge as Mommy."

I was putting something on my face to make it less shiny:

Karis: "Mom, I think you should put extra on your forehead because that is your worst spot. I think it's because it's the highest and the light shines off it."

Thanks Ker! Even my 8 year old notices my shiny face!

Audrey hugged me and said: "Mmmm, you smell good!"

Ariel: "I do!?" (This surprised me since I don't wear any fragrances because they give me migraines.)

Audrey (sighs): "Yeah, you smell like salad, Mmmm!"

If my kids think salad smells good, I must be doing something right!

Tyler: "Come on, Mom! Put on your 'try hard' pants!"

Karis: "The only reason I want to grow up is so I can have an iPhone and babies that I can snuggle and put to bed but I don't want to deal with like money or cleaning the house but I do want to have a mansion but I'll just pay someone to clean that!"

#thevisionoflittleones

Audrey was saying something that Karis didn't like:

Karis: "Audrey, stop! You are only 11 and I am a grown woman!"

She's 8.

Karis: "Mom how old are you again?"

Ariel: "37."

Karis: "WHAT!? You don't look that old! You look like college...no, like the age right before college but the absolute youngest you could look is 15 but you look more like 17. I mean what do you DO to look so young?"

I was looking for something on Netflix:

Karis: "Mommy, just TRY *Phinius and Ferb*. You might like it! You might get addicted like me! Just binge watch it!"

Karis: "I SO just wanna order something! I wanna order a toy or SOMETHING! It just feels SO good to get a package! When a package comes I'm like YAY, a package!"

#iknowthefeeling #girlsaresomuchfun

I was having a semi-serious conversation with the kids. When we were done I asked, "Does anyone else have anything on their mind they want to say?" Connor said: "Nope! I just like the color blue."

Tyler (has three ref jobs today): "Connor, don't waste your day! Go to some friends' house! Soon you will have a jcb and your life will be boring like me!"

Tyler: "Ugh, Mom! Why are you such a handful!?"

Connor: "Mom, we paid off our van so don't worry about if we crash it or anything!"

Connor was sitting on my lap and Audrey came and started bothering him.

Connor: "Everything was fine until YOU got here!"

Audrey: "Everything wasn't fine UNTIL I got here!"

Connor: "Everything wasn't fine my whole entire life because you were born before me!"

Karis: "Mommy, can I live with you for the rest of my life even when I'm married and have kids?"

229

Ariel: "Of course!"

Matt: "Wait, what!? Mommy, didn't discuss this with me!"

Karis: "Mommy, if Daddy says no can you make him?"

Tyler: "I remember growing up we used to...."

Connor: "You still ARE growing up!"

Tyler: "No, I mean when I was a kid."

Connor: "You still ARE a kid!"

Tyler: "No, I mean when I was little."

Connor: "You still ARE little!"

Tyler: "It's so much easier and relaxing to just be negative and critical. It's HARD being positive, takes so much work, ya know?!"

Tyler (13) trying to get out of math: "Mom I'll have talk time with you and snuggle with you!"

#staystrongmommystaystrong!

Tyler: "Isn't it funny that we know more than Mom and Dad and we're only kids!?"

Karis: "Well, we don't know more SCHOOL stuff...because Mom has to teach us...."

Tyler: "Yeah, but like common sense stuff...I mean they just laugh at each other and no one else thinks it's funny!"

Karis (with a BIG sigh): "I just want to get a job. Why don't they have any good jobs for 8 year olds!? They should make a Chic-fil-A where little kids can work...and a little road with little cars so when you can't take me somewhere I can drive myself! I mean seriously!"

Tyler: "Mom if we drive you crazy it's because of mistakes you've made in the past with parenting!"

#tellitlikeitisTy!! #wisefunnyman

Karis: "Mommy, how did you get so pretty other than that's how God made you?"

#howdidyougetsosweet!?

Ariel: "My hair still smells like smoke from the bonfire last night!

Karis: "Let me smell. Mmmm, smells like steak!"

Karis: "You know what would make you an even better, Mommy? I mean, you are still the best Mommy in the world but you know what will make you an even better one? Getting us a dog!"

#noway #illsettleforsecondbest

2017 Quotes

Ariel: "Connor, did you learn anything at Mommy's Juice Plus event last night?

Con: "Yeah, to do the shed 10, so I can have lots and lots of Juice Plus shakes!"

Connor: "Mom! Can I have a chocolate Juice Plus bar and flood my body with antioxidants and whole food nutrition!?"

2018 Quotes

Tyler: "I just want freedom! I mean, I know you and Dad are new to this parenting thing but I'm the child who has to deal with it."

Karis:"Mom! What if you were one of those people who didn't have kids! Then I wouldn't exist and I LOVE existing!"

Tyler: "Mom, look, I look so much younger!"

Ariel: "Ummm, Ummm...."

Tyler: "I shaved my peach fuzz! Look how much younger I look!"

Karis: "I get a house for free, food for free, gymnastics for free, a free harp, free music lessons, it's a great life!"

Ariel: "Connor, stop bothering Karis!"

Connor: "I'm not! I'm just having fun!"

Tyler on Ariel taking pictures: "Oh look, remember that time when Mom was taking pictures of us doing this...and that other time Mom was taking pictures of us doing that...and, oh yeah, look at that time Mom was taking pictures of us doing that...."

In the middle of church, Karis leans over and pulls a five out of her purse: "I'll give you this if we can leave early?" Slides over a 10, "This?"

Karis: "Mom, does my bow look OK?"

Ariel: "Yes, you always look beautiful."

K: "Mom, don't be my mother! Just be a normal person!"

Karis: "If the hurricane is the worst Friday, then Thursday night I'm making sure all my electronics are full battery."

Karis to Ariel: "I want you to be happy but I want myself to be happy more."

Ariel had to wake up one morning. K pushed her away and said, "I'm going back to my dream. It was sooo good. It was about a really yummy dessert!"

Karis: "Mom, you can either get me a pet or have another baby, OK?"

Ariel: "Karis, why are you making such a mess?"

Karis: "Because I'm pretending I'm in one of those cooking shows!"

References:

This is by no means an exhaustive list of all the supplements and medications that I was on. In addition, everyone's body is different and needs/responds differently to different treatments and medication. Please work with your doctor to find the best treatment for you.

https://arielselwyn.juiceplus.com Here you will find raw, vine ripened fruits and vegetables in capsule and chewable form.

https://arielselwyn.norwex.biz/ Here you will find safe, chemical-free cleaning products for your home and office.

http://www.optimalhealthdimensions.com/ Dr. Zackrison's website.

http://www.sterlingfamilypractice.com/ Dr. Fletcher's website.

https://www.jefferson.edu/university/jmc/departments/neurology/programs/headache.html/ The Jefferson Headache Center with Dr Marmura.

https://atlasspineartscenter.com/ Dr. Lim, orthogonal chiropractor.

https://suzycohen.com/ Dr. Suzy Cohen, ways to naturally heal without medication, particularly focused on the thyroid, adrenals and headaches.

https://www.mercola.com/ Dr. Mercola, the cutting edge of alternative health, where I bought my grounding mat and probiotics.

https://www.psychologytoday.com/us/therapists/kathleen-e-hanagan-alexandria-va/195280/ Kathleen Hanagan, Brain Spotting.

https://www.tuckerpsychiatric.com/ Dr Spainer, the psychiatrist who put me on Lexapro (long term) and Lamictal for a short time.

https://www.drberg.com/ Dr Berg. Key in getting my husband's health back on track.

https://www.ozonegenerator.com/ where I bought my at home ozone generator

Squatty Potty and Mag07 can both be found at Amazon.com

NAET: Nambudripad's Allergy Elimination Techniques, also known as NAET, is a non-invasive, drug free, natural solution to alleviate allergies of all types. It does so by using a variety of testing procedures and then balancing the body's energy. There are a variety of treatment procedures including acupuncture/acupressure.

NAET uses Muscle Response Testing (MRT) to confirm the presence of allergic reactivity. NAET offers an alternative solution to eliminating allergic conditions by balancing the body and mind.

EFT: Emotional freedom technique (EFT) is an alternative treatment for physical and emotional pain and distress. It's also more commonly known as tapping. People who use EFT believe tapping the body can create a balance in your energy system and therefore relieve the emotional or physical pain. The tapping is methodical in nature and is around specific points on the face, hands and under the arm. There are also certain things to say while tapping that an experienced EFT therapist can help with.

https://www.askdrsears.com/ Great website for health, especially for kids and where I received my health coach certification

http://www.drmitraray.com/ Great source for health information, Dr Mitra Ray

Other helpful health websites: www.amymeyersmd.com www.draxe.com www.drhyman.com/

https://www.abeka.com/homeschool/ our homeschool curriculum

ATP energy– similar to ATP Ignite but capsule form and no caffeine

ALA– Alfa lipoic acid

Resveratrol– powerful antioxidant

Tumeric – spice known for it's health benefits including being an anti-inflammatory

CoQ10- *Powerful antioxidant*; our bodies naturally produce this but production decreases as we age

Astaxanthan-Powerful anti-inflammatory; naturally found in things like algae; gives salmon it's pink pigment

ATP Ignite – comes in a powder packet to mix into water, contains electrolytes, antioxidants, caffeine, B vitamins, trace minerals, amino acids, herbs

Bio Cleanse Plus– GI and liver support, Shake meal

Resveratrol– anti-aging antioxidant known to help with pain, especially headaches

Milk Thistle– cleanses the liver

Serretia– 99.99% pure Serratiopeptidase, proteolytic enzyme

Probiotics– always used Dr. Mercola's

Saccrimyces Boulardi– prebiotic

L-Glutamine– heals and seals the gut lining

Cortisol Management– levels out cortisol levels, helps sleep at night and helps with stress levels

Simalase Lipo– digestive enzyme

Electrolytes- Helps with hydration; must stay balanced in the body for maximum health: sodium, calcium, potassium, chloride, phosphate, and magnesium

Argentyn 23– immune support

CBD oil– used for many reasons. I was trying it to see if it would help with the headaches.

Wendy Roberts, NP at Dr. Zackrison's office provided the description for the following.

Moon Pearls- Chinese herbal blend for hormone ba ance including support for thyroid, adrenals, ovaries and pituitary

IG 26 Powder- immunoglobulins to support gut lining and the immune system; similar to colostrum but stronger

KLS- herbal blend for support and cleansing of the kidneys, liver and spleen

Scrofulara- liver support

Phonphorus Oligo- micronized phosphorus replacement

Potassium Oligo- micronized potassium replacement

Mestenon- modulates receptors for acetylcholine at the neuromuscular receptor. Helps with fluctuant blood pressure seen in POTS off label, but is used in diseases like myasthenia gravis on label.

Cupermine- old drug used for RA. Modifies joint inflammation.

Eliquis- anticoagulant

BiliBile- support for bile production and bile flow

CEDSA, ASSYRA, ZYTO, EVOX- used for electrodermal indication of imbalance in the body.

About the Author

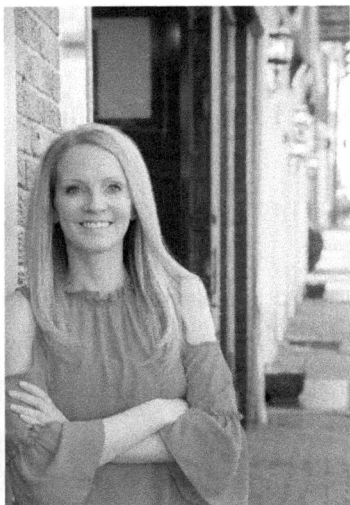

Ariel graduated from the University of Mary Washington in 2001. She married her husband, Matthew, in 2002 and they have four children together. Ariel taught mathematics at Brooke Point High School before their first child was born. She stayed home with their four children for 15 years before going back to work for the Navy as a Configuration Management Specialist.

She is also a certified hydrotherapist and certified health coach. In addition, she works part time for the Juice Plus company and is a co-author of *Dust to Salvation,* which will be released in March 2020.

Ariel decided to write *Though the Mountains Be Shaken* for those who are striving to be the person they envisioned in the face of life's challenges. In this book, Ariel tries to live up to the quote, "I want to inspire others. I want them to look at me and say, 'Because of you, I didn't give up.' "

You can find more information about Ariel on her website, arielselwyn.com, or on Instagram @ariel.selwyn

www.ingramcontent.com/pod-product-compliance
Lightning Source LLC
Chambersburg PA
CBHW060315030426
42336CB00011B/1060